Posttraumatic Embitterment Disorder

Posttraumatic Embitterment Disorder

Michael Linden
Max Rotter
Kai Baumann
Barbara Lieberei

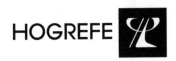
HOGREFE

Library of Congress Cataloging in Publication

is available via the Library of Congress Marc Database under the
LC Control Number 2006928921

Library and Archives Canada Cataloguing in Publication

Posttraumatic embitterment disorder: definition, evidence, diagnosis,
treatment / Michael Linden ... [et al.].
ISBN 0-88937-344-2
    1. Adjustment disorders. 2. Stress tolerance (Psychology) I. Linden,
Michael
RC455.4.S87P67 2006   152.4   C2006-903420-6

© 2007 by Hogrefe & Huber Publishers

PUBLISHING OFFICES
USA: Hogrefe & Huber Publishers, 875 Massachusetts Avenue, 7th Floor,
                  Cambridge, MA 02139
                  Phone (866) 823-4726, Fax (617) 354-6875; E-mail info@hhpub.com
EUROPE: Hogrefe & Huber Publishers, Rohnsweg 25, 37085 Göttingen, Germany
                  Phone +49 551 49609-0, Fax +49 551 49609-88, E-mail hh@hhpub.com

SALES & DISTRIBUTION
USA: Hogrefe & Huber Publishers, Customer Services Department,
                  30 Amberwood Parkway, Ashland, OH 44805
                  Phone (800) 228-3749, Fax (419) 281-6883, E-mail custserv@hhpub.com
EUROPE: Hogrefe & Huber Publishers, Rohnsweg 25, 37085 Göttingen, Germany
                  Phone +49 551 49609-0, Fax +49 551 49609-88, E-mail hh@hhpub.com

OTHER OFFICES
CANADA: Hogrefe & Huber Publishers, 1543 Bayview Avenue, Toronto, Ontario M4G 3B5
SWITZERLAND: Hogrefe & Huber Publishers, Länggass-Strasse 76, CH-3000 Bern 9

Hogrefe & Huber Publishers
Incorporated and registered in the State of Washington, USA, and in Göttingen, Lower Saxony, Germany

Printed and bound in the USA
ISBN-10: 0-88937-344-2
ISBN-13: 978-0-88937-344-0

"Men are not disturbed by things but by the views
which they take of them"

(Epictetus, *Enchiridion*)

Preface

It is generally accepted in clinical medicine that stressful life events can impair psychological and somatic functioning (Van der Kolk et al. 1994; Van der Kolk et al. 1996; Paykel, 2001a; Paykel, 2001b). In the international classification systems ICD-10 (World Health Organization – WHO, 1992) and DSM-IV (American Psychiatric Association – APA, 1994) such disorders are grouped together as adjustment disorders.

An increase of such reactive disorders was observed in the wake of German reunification, as 17 million inhabitants of the former GDR were faced with re-organizing their biographies, with up to one third of the population still expressing feelings of having been let down a decade later (Schwarzer & Jerusalem, 1994). However, no differences in the rate of mental disorders in East and West were found immediately after the fall of the Berlin wall (Dehlinger & Ortmann, 1992; Achberger, Linden, & Benkert, 1999; Wittchen, Müller, Pfister, Winter, & Schmidtkunz, 1999; Hillen, Schaub, Hiestermann, Kirschner, & Robra, 2000). Yet ten years later, patients presented with severe psychological reactions to negative changes in their personal biographies, which, for several reasons, could be diagnosed neither as posttraumatic stress disorder (PTSD) nor adjustment disorder nor depressive disorder according to the definitions of ICD-10 or DSM-IV. Instead, these patients showed distinct and characteristic psychopathological features, a marked course, and special treatment needs.

This increase in pathological reactions to critical life events in the aftermath of German reunification made it possible to recognize a distinct reaction type with its own etiology and psychopathological characteristics. This reaction type is universal and frequently seen in patients who have had to cope with events of personal injustice, humiliation, frustration, and helplessness. Within minutes, such events can lead to a change from perfect health to prolonged down-heartedness, hopelessness, embitterment, and impairment in all areas of life. This reaction type can best be described as 'posttraumatic embitterment disorder' (PTED).

PTED is a reactive disorder triggered by an exceptional, though normal negative life event such as conflict in the workplace, unemployment, death of a relative, divorce, severe illness, or experience of loss or separation. The common feature of such events is that they are experienced as unjust, as a personal insult, and that psychologically there is a violation of basic beliefs and values. The central psychopathological response pattern in PTED is a prolonged feeling of embitterment.

To further study PTED, a research project was initiated within the Research Group Psychosomatic Rehabilitation at the Charité in Berlin and the Department of Behavioral Medicine and Psychosomatics at the Rehabilitation Center

Seehof, Teltow/Berlin, financed by the German pension fund (Deutsche Rent-enversicherung), as many of these patients end up taking prolonged sick leave and early retirement. The objective of the project was to better delineate the clinical features of this syndrome, to develop diagnostic criteria, and to open avenues for treatment. This first monograph on posttraumatic embitterment disorder gives a comprehensive overview of the recent developments in PTED research.

The first part of this book gives an overview of the theoretical background of stress and stress reactions in clinical research. Chapter 1.1. describes how stress reactions to life events and their role in the development of illness found entrance into the psychiatric and psychological nomenclature. Different conceptualizations of stress and life events as stressors and etiological agents are discussed. In addition, methodological aspects of life events research and findings on the connection between life stress and psychiatric disorders are presented. Chapter 1.2. introduces the diagnostic categories of the present international classification systems ICD-10 (WHO, 1992) and DSM-IV (APA, 1994) that refer to reactive disorders. The definition of adjustment disorders, findings on epidemiology and etiology, as well as different treatment approaches are presented. Moreover, the role of adjustment disorders in clinical practice is analyzed, and PTSD is introduced as an example of a well-defined reactive disorder. Chapter 1.3. presents the theoretical concept of PTED as a special form of adjustment disorder, and important aspects of the syndrome are out-lined in detail. Chapter 1.4. discusses psychological and etiological models. In particular, "violation of basic beliefs" and "lack of wisdom" are introduced as possible etiological factors for PTED. Chapter 1.5. describes the field of wisdom research and illustrates an approach to operationalizing and measuring wisdom-related performance.

The second part of the book summarizes empirical data on PTED derived from a number of studies on the subject. Chapter 2.1. outlines data on the psychopathological and emotional profile of patients with PTED. Also, PTED patients are compared with patients with other mental disorders as regards quality and intensity of psychopathological as well as posttraumatic symp-toms. Chapter 2.2. presents empirically derived diagnostic criteria according to the rules of the DSM-IV and a diagnostic interview for PTED. Chapter 2.3. describes a self-rating scale for PTED. This instrument was developed to measure symptom severity in diagnosed cases of PTED. Data on a principle component analysis of the scale, internal consistency, test-retest reliability, and convergent and discriminant validity are presented. Chapter 2.4. reports data on the epidemiology of PTED in clinical and nonclinical populations. Chapter 2.5. discusses etiological concepts and vulnerability factors with a focus on the psychology of wisdom.

The third part of the book presents first concepts for treatment of PTED. After discussing traditional treatment approaches for reactive disorders and their application in PTED (chapter 3.1.), "wisdom therapy," a treatment approach specifically developed for PTED, is introduced in chapter 3.2. A detailed treatment guideline for PTED is presented.

The authors hope that this first monograph on PTED will help to introduce and explain this disorder. Patients with mental problems of this kind are seriously ill, they suffer personally and also put severe burdens on family members, coworkers, or friends. They are severely impaired in most areas of life. They are undoubtedly in need of help. But they typically reject help, they do not come to ask for treatment, and if they are seen in psychiatric and psychotherapeutic services they are often misunderstood and wrongly diagnosed. In many cases, treatment ends in failure. Therefore more research is urgently needed. The authors are happy to share their instruments and theoretical and clinical knowledge with all who are interested in working in this field.

List of Tables

Table 1. Case vignette of PTED. 19
Table 2. Research diagnostic criteria for PTED. 23
Table 3. General criteria outlining the nature of wisdom derived
from cultural-historical analysis (Baltes & Staudinger,
2000, p. 135) 36
Table 4. Five criteria characterizing wisdom and wisdom-related
performance (Staudinger & Baltes, 1996b, p. 747) 40
Table 5. Wisdom-related task with examples of extreme
responses (abbreviated) (Baltes & Staudinger, 2000,
p. 136) 41
Table 6. Dimensions of cognitive and emotional wisdom-related
expertise. 47
Table 7. Sociodemographic data of PTED and control patients 54
Table 8. Diagnostic spectrum according to the MINI standardized
interview ($N = 100$) 55
Table 9. SCL-90-R, Bern Embitterment Questionnaire, and
IES-R scores. 60
Table 10. Clinical diagnostic criteria for PTED. 63
Table 11. Research diagnostic criteria for PTED. 65
Table 12. The diagnostic interview for PTED 70
Table 13. Spearman Rho Coefficients (time interval of 6–8 days),
rotated factor solution and within-group correlations
with the discriminant function 75
Table 14. Intercorrelations of the PTED Scale with concurrent
validity measures assessed with data from the PTED
sample ($n = 48$). 79
Table 15. Sociodemographic data of the train sample for women
and men ($N = 158$) 82
Table 16. Sociodemographic data and occupational situation of
the GP sample ($N = 221$) 84
Table 17. Set of linear nonorthogonal contrasts. 94
Table 18. List of fictitious life problems that can be used in
wisdom therapy 112

List of Figures

Figure 1. Duration of PTED ($n = 48$). 58

Figure 2. Psychopathological spectrum in connection with the
critical event ($n = 48$) 58

Figure 3. Emotional spectrum in connection with the
critical event ($n = 48$) 59

Figure 4. Frequency distribution of the unselected inpatient
sample for each item of the PTED Scale ($N=100$) 74

Figure 5. Mean scores of both subsamples of the Seehof sample
for each item of the PTED Scale ($N = 96$) 78

Figure 6. Frequency distribution (in %) of the train sample
($N = 158$) for the five-point answer categories of each
item on the PTED Scale 83

Figure 7. Frequency distribution (in %) of the GP sample ($N = 221$)
for the five-point answer categories of each item on the
PTED Scale. 87

Figure 8. Frequency distributions of four different samples on the
PTED Scale (mean total scores) 88

Figure 9. Wisdom-related performance of the PTED sample
and the control group ($N = 98$) in connection to
fictitious life problems on the nine wisdom scales
(pretest assessment). 93

Figure 10. Wisdom-related performance of the PTED sample
and the control group ($N = 98$) in connection to a
personal life problem on the nine wisdom scales
(pretest assessment). 93

Figure 11. Mean total scores of each group for the pre- and
posttest in the fictitious problem condition. 95

Figure 12. Mean total scores of each group for the pre- and
posttest in the personal problem condition 96

Figure 13. Wisdom-related performance of the subsamples
of the PTED sample in connection to a personal life
problem on the nine wisdom scales (posttest assessment). . . . 97

Table of Contents

Preface. vii
List of Tables. xi
List of Figures. xiii

1. Conceptual Issues. 1
1.1 Reactions to Stress and Life Events. 3
1.2 Adjustment and Reactive Disorders. 11
1.3 Posttraumatic Embitterment Disorder (PTED) 17
1.4 Basic Beliefs and PTED. 28
1.5 Wisdom and PTED 33

2. Empirical Evidence. 49
2.1 The Psychopathology of PTED 53
2.2 Diagnostic Interview and Criteria for PTED 63
2.3 The PTED Self-Rating Scale 72
2.4 The Epidemiology of PTED 81
2.5 Wisdom and Activation of Wisdom-Related Knowledge in PTED . . 91

3. Treatment Perspectives 99
3.1 Cognitive Behavior Therapy for PTED 101
3.2 Wisdom Therapy 107
3.3 A Case Vignette 116

4. References 119

5. Appendix 137
    PTED Self-Rating Scale 139
    Diagnostic Core Interview and Algorithm for PTED 140
    Clinical Semi-Standardized Diagnostic Interview for PTED 142
    Wisdom Rating Scale 147
    Wisdom Training Outline. 150

1. Conceptual Issues

1.1 Reactions to Stress and Life Events

Early concepts of stress and psychological disorders

In attempting to understand the antecedents of psychopathology, theorists historically have sought explanations from two spheres. On the one hand, the belief has long been held that individuals who develop a psychiatric disorder differ premorbidly from those who do not. Such differences were thought to be constitutional in origin (e.g., Beard, 1881). On the other hand, the belief has also long been held that stress is an important factor in the development of psychological disturbances (e.g., Hawkes, 1857). Stress reactions and coping with threatening events have been at the center of research since the early days of psychology (Reck, 2001; Linden, 2003). Examples of early terms for stress-related illnesses were "railway spine," "psychogenic or reactive depression," "traumatic neurosis," or "abnormal psychological reaction" (Jaspers, 1973; Freud, 1999; Van der Kolk, Weisath & Van der Hart, 2000). A better recognition of the nature and consequences of battle stress followed the experience of the two World Wars, and terms like "shellshock" or "combat neurosis" emerged (Maercker, 2003).

An understanding of the impact of negative life events which lie more in the realm of common experience on the development of mental illnesses was slower to develop (Paykel, 2001b). In the following, research on life events which addresses possible effects of stressful everyday experiences will be reviewed and presented.

Life event research

The subject of life event research are the effects of life events on behavior, experience, and mental or physical health of the individual(s) in question (Filipp, 1995). There is common consent that relevant changes in life are associated with certain demands, which request specific processing, adjustment, and orientation performances (Dittmann, 1991). Petermann (1995; p.53) defines relevant (or critical) life events as a grouping of favorable or unfavorable social circumstances that are psychologically relevant, and which may be verified by their effects (stress, illness). A more general definition has been put forward by Filipp (1995; p. 23), who characterizes life events as changes in the (social) life situation that demand adaptation behavior of the individual concerned.

Filipp (1995) differentiates two major theoretical branches within the field of life event research: The clinical psychological approach, which examines psychosocial causes of physical and mental illnesses, and the developmental psychological approach, which conceptualizes life events as a precondition for developmental change.

The foundation for systematic experimental research on the pathological effects of stressful events was laid by Cannon (1929). His detailed observations of bodily changes caused by stressful conditions and strong emotions provided a necessary link in the argument that stressful events can prove harmful (Dohrenwend & Dohrenwend, 1974a). Thereafter, a vast body of research evolved based on the hypothesis that stressful life events play a role in the etiology of various somatic and psychiatric disorders. This line of research can best be described as clinical life event research.

The early years of clinical life event research were accompanied by a vigorous debate on the causative effect of life events between those supporting a psychological causation of disorders, and those who saw the causes of psychiatric disorders in constitutional, genetic, and biological factors. This polarization in psychiatry has now been put to rest for the most part, as the place of life events in the causative chain of illness development has become generally accepted (Paykel, 2001b).

An early major influence on clinical life event research lay in the views of Adolph Meyer (1951). With his invention of the "life chart," a device for organizing medical data as a dynamic biography, Meyer (1951) emphasized that various life events within common experience could form an important part of the etiology of a disorder. That is to say, different kinds of events can contribute to the development of an illness, even events that are welcomed, e.g., marriage or winning the lottery.

This view was supported by the findings of Selye (1956), who, in a series of animal studies, observed that a variety of stimulus events (e.g., heat, cold, toxic agents) applied intensely and over a long period of time are capable of producing common effects, meaning not specific to either stimulus event. Based on these findings Selye claimed that all organisms show a nonspecific response to adverse stimulation, no matter what the actual situation is. This response follows a typical three-stage pattern, called the "general adaptation syndrome" (GAS).

Adaptation and life events

According to Selye, the organism initially defends itself against adverse stimulation by activating the sympathetic nervous system (*alarm reaction*). This first reaction to a stressor mobilizes the body for the "fight or flight" reaction. In many cases, the stress episode is managed during the alarm reaction stage. However, if the adverse stimulation continues over a longer period of time, the organism moves on to the *resistance stage,* in which it adapts more or less successfully to the persistent stress. In this stage, the symptoms of the alarm reaction disappear though, according to Selye, an organism in this stage does not function well. Its immune system is impaired, and some typical "diseases of adaptation" (e.g., cardiovascular diseases) develop. Finally, if the stress does not subside, the organism enters the *exhaustion stage.* The adaptation resources are depleted, and breakdown occurs. Irreversible tissue damage occurs, and if the stimulation persists, the organism dies.

In reference to the work of Meyer and Selye, Holmes and Masuda (1974) postulated that life events lower "bodily resistance" and enhance the probability of disease occurrence by evoking dysfunctional adaptive efforts by the human organism that are faulty in kind and duration. This claim initiated a new approach to the investigation of the psychosocial causes of disease. Central to this approach is the assumption that the human capacity to adapt to life changes is limited. Thus, the confrontation with an accumulation of life-changing events within a certain time can have pathological consequences (Filipp, 1995). In this view, life events produce challenges to the organism regardless of their specific (e.g., positive or negative) quality, and therefore increase illness susceptibility.

In accordance with this view, Rahe, Meyer, Smith, Kjar and Holmes (1964) demonstrated that a cluster of social events requiring change and adjustment in ongoing life were significantly associated with the time of illness onset. Subsequently, the *Social Readjustment Rating Scale* (SRRS) was introduced by Holmes and Rahe (1967). The SRRS is an early attempt to quantify the challenge (stress) of specific critical life events to the organism,[1] by assigning predefined values, called life change units, to 43 critical life events (e.g., vacation, jail term, Christmas). It was assumed that the average amount of adaptive effort necessary to cope with an event would be a useful indicator of the severeness of such an event (Schwarzer & Schulz, 2002). By asking for the intensity and length of time which is necessary to accommodate to a life event, independent of the desirability of this event, "change from the existing state" became the pivotal factor and not the psychological meaning of the event, e.g., associated emotions or social desirability (Holms & Rahe, 1967).

Although criticized for methodological shortcomings, the Social Readjustment Rating Scale had a powerful influence on the field of clinical life event

---

[1] An earlier attempt to quantify life stress was the *Schedule of Recent Experiences* (SRE) (Hawkins, Davies, & Holmes, 1957). The development of the SRRS was based on the SRE. The SRRS is the more refined and better-known instrument.

research by introducing a structured list of stressful life events and a method of stress quantification. A number of interviews and self-report questionnaires have subsequently been developed to obtain information about recent life events. Today, the most prominent and frequently used questionnaires in clinical live event research are the *Interview for Recent Life Events* (Paykel, 1983) and the *Life Events and Difficulties Schedule* (Brown & Harris, 1978).[2]

Specificity of stressors

Investigations on the effects of specific life events and new findings in the field of endocrinology (Mason, 1975) challenged the assumption of an unspecific impact of critical life events (Holmes & Rahe, 1967). Although the founding fathers of life event research saw "readjustment" as the core feature for the promotion of nonspecific vulnerability to virtually any form of illness, recent research indicates that more specific qualities of life experiences are also of importance (Monroe & Simons, 1991).

In a review of 27 studies, Paykel and Copper (1992) found that bereavement and separation showed a strong connection to depression onset (Reck, 2001). Brown, Bifulco, and Harris (1987) found a connection between depression onset and life events which trigger the experience of role conflict and/or high obligations. For the development of anxiety disorders, threatening events seem to be of special relevance (Finlay-Jones & Brown, 1981; Finlay-Jones, 1989). In contrast to this, no influence of positive life events on the onset of illness has been found (Reck, 2001), and it has not been possible to empirically verify the so-called "depression by success" (e.g., Reimer, 1995). These findings speak against the concept of an unspecific impact of life events and the importance of a general life change factor as suggested by Holmes and Masuda (1974).

The diathesis–stress model

Another theoretical approach in clinical life event research are diathesis-stress models (Reck, 2001), which focus on the interaction of predisposing diathesis and precipitating environmental stress factors. Diathesis can be understood as a tendency to react in a certain way to environmental circumstances. It comprises physiological as well as psychological aspects. An essential feature of diathesis-stress models is the assumption that the diathesis (or the vulnerability) has no consequences as long as no stressful event occurs.

---

[2] For a comprehensive overview see Reck (2001).

Diathesis-stress models allow the formulation of hypotheses about the probability of illness occurrence. A prominent example for a diathesis-stress model is Beck's (1967, 1983) cognitive theory of depression. Beck assumes that latent depressiogenic schemata are present in individuals vulnerable to depression. However, without the occurrence of negative events (the stress), individuals who possess depressiogenic schemata (the diathesis) are no more likely to become depressed than individuals who do not posses such schemata (see also Abela & Alessandro, 2002). Brown and Harris (1978) found that vulnerability factors for the development of depression in women are: lack of a trusting partnership or marriage, loss of mother before the age of 11, three or more children at home, or lack of a task beyond the household. The existence of one or more of these factors is thought to increase the probability of depression if a stressful life event occurs.

The diathesis-stress model (stress triggers diathesis) was extended by Monroe and Simons (1991), who proposed three alternatives of diathesis-stress interactions:

a) Both the diathesis and the stress together constitute a necessary condition for illness onset. Neither is sufficient by itself.

b) The only necessary factor for illness onset is the diathesis. Stress is either a minor factor, a result of the diathesis' expression, or simply a consequence of the emerging illness.

c) The only necessary factor for illness onset is life stress, the diathesis only increases the likelihood of the stressor to occur.

These different aspects of diathesis-stress interactions represent different approaches to how the interaction between endogenous and exogenous factors and their contribution to illness development can be conceptualized.

Transactional concepts

The clinical psychological/psychiatric perspective on life event research, which, in reference to Meyer and Selye, focuses on the characteristics of life events and the respective quantity of stress that is triggered by these events, has been criticized by health and developmental psychologists (Filipp, 1995; Krohne, 2001; Schwarzer & Schulz, 2002).[3]

These critics claim that the amount of stress cannot be determined by the objective nature of the stressor alone. In looking only at this, individual differences in perception and interpretation of the same kind of event are neglected

---

[3] For a good example of the clinical psychological/psychiatric perspective see Dohrenwend & Dohrenwend (1974).

(Schwarzer & Schulz, 2002). This criticism emphasizes the importance of subjective interpretation of the stressor for the experience of stress. A major proponent of this conceptualization of stress is Lazarus (1966), who defines stress as a particular relationship ("transaction") between the individual and the environment that is appraised by the individual as being taxing or exceeding his or her resources and endangering her or his well-being. A major advantage of this concept is that it can explain individual differences in quality, intensity, and duration of experienced stress in environments that are objectively equal. By integrating person variables, such as commitments, personal health or beliefs into the conceptualization of stress, the focus is moved away from the objective nature of stressors to a transactional process between the individual and his or her environment, with both of these components exerting a reciprocal influence on each other (Schwarzer & Schulz, 2002). In this vein, life events are not only conceptualized as possible etiologic agents for illness, but also as tasks that challenge the individual and can further his or her development (Filipp, 1995).

Many factors are involved in determining the type of reaction to a certain stressor. The meaning of stress is affected by "modifiers," such as ego strength, support systems, and prior mastery (Cohen, 1981). Schwarzer & Schulze (2002) state that societal structures as well as cultural norms and values largely determine the way individuals respond to stress. Several social and personal constructs have been proposed to explain individual stress responses: *Social support* (Schwarzer & Leppin, 1991), *sense of coherence* (Antonovsky, 1979), *hardiness* (Kobasa, 1979), *self-efficacy* (Bandura, 1977), or *optimism* (Scheier & Carver, 1992). As a consequence, many authors have stressed that the vulnerability of the individual (e.g., ego strengths, support system, self-efficacy, sense of coherence, control over the stressors and desirability of the event) needs to be assessed to ascertain the impact of the situation on the individual (Strain et al. 1999).

In addition to subjective interpretations, variables like gender, culture, ethnicity, and age have been discussed to explain differences in the experience of stressful life events (Schwarzer & Schulz, 2002). Apart from the objective impact of an event, societal structures, cultural norms, and personal values also determine how individuals respond to an incident. Gillard and Paton (1999), for example, found that religious denomination had an impact on vulnerability. Furthermore, there is ample evidence for gender differences in response to stressful life events (e.g., Karanci, Alkan, Sucuoglu, & Aksit, 1999; Ben-Zur, & Zeidner, 1991). Higher situational stress assessment as well as more pronounced stress experience was found among women.[4] Norris, Perilla, Ibañez, and Murphy

---

[4] For a discussion of possible reasons for this gender difference see Schwarzer and Schulz (2002).

(2001) found that women from Mexico were more likely to meet the criteria for PTSD following a hurricane than women from the United States, suggesting that cultural differences influence the way traumatic events are experienced.

Findings on the effect of age on coping with adverse stimulation are rare and contradictory. Some found a decrease of coping abilities with increasing age (e.g., Toukmanian, Jadaa, & Lawless, 2000; Cwikel, & Rozovski, 1998), while others found older people were more resistant to stress (e.g., Ben-Zur, & Zeidner, 1991; Muthny, Gramus, Dutton, & Stegie, 1987).

Another factor that needs to be taken into account is the possible additive impact of a stressor. A recent minor stress superimposed on a previous major stress that has no observable effect on its own may have a cataclysmic effect due to its additive impact. In this regard, the model of a single stressor imping-ing on an undisturbed individual to cause symptoms at a single point in time appears to be insufficient to account for the many presentations of stress in an individual.

The findings on life events and their effects gathered in the fields of health and developmental psychology show that the conceptualization of life events, as stressors that impinge a quantifiable amount of distress on the organism, is not able to capture the numerous factors which influence the impact and experi-ence of negative life events.

Diathesis-stress models (e.g., Monroe & Simons, 1991) are useful to un-derstand the connections between stressful life events, personal factors, and illness development.[5] Event-specific factors as well as individual (cognitive and biological) factors are taken into account. However, the importance of social resources as well as cultural and societal variables for stress experience is still insufficiently integrated (Reck, 2001).

Problems with the assessment of stressors

Apart from theoretical conceptualizations of negative life events there are also several basic problems with their assessment. The first is the definition of an event as "critical." Due to the fact that "critical" life events are defined by their consequences, every definition of a "critical" event is somewhat circular in nature (Reinecker, 2003).

The second problem is that life event data are typically obtained by retro-spective history taking. Starting from the observable effect (illness), one tries

---

5 For example, Brown & Harris (1989) account for the demand of integrating subjective interpretations of the event by integrating the context in which an event takes place and the personal understanding of an event into their assessment.

to assess preceding critical events. This method has a number of advantages and disadvantages. An advantage of retrospective studies is that they are able to cover a long life-span. Thus, events that happened a long time ago can be assessed. In addition, the retrospective method integrates individual experiences of events. As a result, it gains indicators about individual ways in which critical events are evaluated or experienced (Petermann, 1995). However, there are a number of methodological problems with the retrospective method, concerning reliability and validity of information. Recollection can be subject to distortion of recall, together with (in the psychiatric patient) misperceptions due to mental illness, such as guilt in depression, or paranoid delusions in schizophrenia (Paykel, 2001b). Furthermore, the patient, psychiatric or medical, may attempt to give meaning to and an explanation for an illness and therefore may overemphasize the significance of events which did occur (Paykel, 1974). An additional problem is the elimination of events that are consequences of illness. The patient may experience events, such as job loss, as a result of his or her disorder. Thus, a confusion of independent and dependent variables can occur (Petermann, 1995). However, many disadvantages of the retrospective approach can be limited by using direct interviews and by confining attention to the period prior to the onset of the illness episode (Paykel, 2001b).

In addition to retrospective studies, there are also a number of longitudinal prospective studies. Here, subjects undergoing a specific event are followed up. Events that have been studied in this manner are bereavement (Lichtenstein, Gatz, & Berg, 1998; Chen, Bierhals, Prigerson, Kasl, Mazure, & Jacobs, 1999), loss of employment (Kasl, Gore, & Gore, 1975; Leino-Arjas, Liira, Mtanen, Malmivaara, & Matikainen, 1999), and mastectomy (Maguire, Lee, Bevington, Kuchemann, Cratebee, & Cornell, 1978). However, these studies resulted in no clear outcome and had only little impact on clinical life event research (Paykel, 2001b).

1.2 Adjustment and Reactive Disorders

Stressors and the onset of mental disorders

Since the late 1960s, researchers have documented the influence of stressful life events on a number of psychiatric disorders. It has been shown that life events tend to occur to an extent greater than chance expectation before a variety of psychiatric disorders, including depression, schizophrenia, and anxiety disorders (Paykel, 1974; Finlay-Jones & Brown, 1981; Paykel, 2001b). The effect is moderate in magnitude but varies with disorder. The influence of stressors is less pronounced in schizophrenia than in depression, probably less strong in bipolar affective disorder than in unipolar, and within unipolar depression stronger in first episodes and milder disorders than in severe recurrent disorders (Paykel, 2003). When looking at these findings, one needs to take into account that the revealed connection between life events and psychiatric disorders is correlative only. Nothing can be said about the causal direction and mechanisms of life events on psychiatric disorders on the basis of these findings.

Even though it has been shown that life events are important in determining the onset of an illness, they are not a sufficient explanation. Life events are only one link in a complex multifactorial causative chain. Whether an event is followed by a disorder must be attributed to other modifying factors, both genetic and environmental, ranging from biochemical through personality and coping mechanisms to social experiences, early or recent (Paykel, 2001b).

Adjustment disorders

Exceptions are adjustment or reactive disorders. In international classification systems for mental disorders, such as ICD-10 (WHO, 1992) and DSM-IV (APA, 1994), there are special chapters for disorders which are defined as responses to a variety of causal stressful events, the symptoms representing an adaptation to these stressors or to their continuing effects (Casey, Dorwick, & Wilkinson, 2001). Under the heading of "Reaction to severe stress and adjustment disorders" (F 43), ICD-10 lists: (a) "acute stress reaction" (F 43.0); (b) "posttraumatic stress disorder" (PTSD; F 43.1); and (c) "adjustment disorders" (F 43.2). Furthermore, there is also the category "enduring personality change after catastrophic experience" (F 62.0)[6]. In the DSM-IV, the chapter on adjustment disorders differentiates between "adjustment disorders with predominant depressed mood" (309.0), "anxiety" (309.24), "mixed anxiety and depressed mood" (309.28), "disturbance of conduct" (309.3), and "disturbance of conduct and emotion" (309.4). Further categories are "PTSD" (309.81) and "acute stress disorder" (308.3) that are listed under anxiety disorders.

The adjustment and reactive disorders are unique within the classification systems, as they are diagnoses with a known etiology and in which the etiological agent is central to the diagnosis. This contradicts the concept of a strictly atheoretical and phenomenological approach to the classification of mental disorders (Strain, Newcorn, Fulop, & Sokolyanskaya, 1999). The essential feature of an adjustment disorder is the development of clinically relevant emotional or behavioral symptoms in response to an identifiable psychosocial event that occurs within 3 months after onset of the stressor. The disorder should by definition resolve within 6 months of the termination of the stressor. If the symptoms last longer, the diagnosis should be changed to chronic adjustment disorder (DSM-IV only) or to another Axis I disorder, if the necessary criteria are fulfilled (WHO, 1992; APA, 1994).

In contrast to other DSM-IV and ICD-10 disorders, there is no clear and specific profile of symptoms for adjustment disorders (Strain et al. 1999), which makes this a vague diagnostic category. Also, it is unclear how the concept of 'clinically relevant reaction' can or should be operationalized. The social, emotional, and vocational dysfunctions which indicate the pathological reaction, are qualitatively and quantitatively unspecified. Hence, they lend themselves neither to reliability nor to validity. By the indication that the distress must be greater than would normally be expected from the stressor, the concept of a maladaptive reaction is further confounded by elements of culture. Expectable reactions to an event can differ within specific cultural environments. Gender responses, developmental level differences, and the meaning of events to an individual are all factors that determine an 'expectable' reaction (Strain et al. 1999).

Another important shortcoming of present diagnostic criteria is that no criteria are offered to quantify stressors for adjustment disorders or to assess their effect or meaning for a particular individual at a given time.

---

[6] The diagnostic category of enduring personality change after catastrophic experience (F 62.0) will be discussed in more detail in chapter 1.3.

Posttraumatic Stress Disorder (PTSD)

Among reactive disorders, PTSD and acute stress disorder represent the only subgroups that have gained the status of well-defined disorders in recent years (Marshall, Spitzer, & Liebowitz, 1999; Davidson, Foa, Blank et al. 1996; Fischer & Riedesser 1999). Acute stress reactions and PTSD both develop in response to exceptionally threatening experiences, but the former subsides within days and the latter is more protracted (Casey et al. 2001).

PTSD is defined by exposure to a traumatic event in which a person experiences, witnesses, or is confronted with the threat of death, serious injury, or a threat to one's own physical integrity resulting in intense fear, helplessness, or horror (WHO, 1992). Examples are war experience, rape, or car accidents (Kulka, Schlenger, Fairbank, Hough, Jordan, Marmar, & Weiss, 1990; Fullerton, McCarroll, Ursano, & Wright, 1992; Blanchard, Hickling, Buckley, Taylor, Vollmer, & Loos, 1996). Such experiences can lead to recurrent recollections of the event, i.e., intrusive thoughts, which cause re-experience of the traumatic arousal and anxiety and can result in the development of avoidance behavior.

PTSD can be understood as a special form of anxiety disorder, in which the initial confrontation with an unconditioned stimulus leads to an unconditioned panic reaction. This results in further panic recurrences mediated either by respective memories and cognitions or by renewed confrontation with conditioned stimuli. Avoidance and phobic behavior can be understood as negative reinforcement.

Epidemiology and recognition of adjustment disorders

Although the definition of adjustment disorders is vague and insufficient they are nevertheless frequent disorders. Andreasen and Wasek (1980) observed that 5% of an inpatient and outpatient sample were labeled as having adjustment disorders. Fabrega, Mezzich, and Mezzich (1987) reported that 2.3% of a sample of patients at a walk-in clinic met criteria for adjustment disorders, with no other diagnoses on Axis I or Axis II; 20% had a diagnosis of adjustment disorders when patients with other Axis I diagnoses were also included. In general hospital psychiatric consultation populations, adjustment disorders were diagnosed in 21.5% (Popkin, Callies, Allan Colón, Eduardo, & Stiebel, 1990), 18.5% (Foster & Oxman, 1994), and 11.5% (Snyder, Strain, & Wolf, 1990) of patients, respectively. Snyder, Strain, and Wolf (1990) found that adjustment disorders are the most common diagnosis in primary care.

Treatment of adjustment disorders

The treatment of adjustment disorders refers primarily to psychotherapeutic measures that help to reduce the impact of the stressor, enhance coping with the stressor, activate support systems, and maximize adaptation (Strain et al. 1999). One can differentiate four main intervention methods that are utilized for the treatment of adjustment disorder.

Cognitive interventions aim at modifying beliefs, expectations, assumptions, and styles of thinking. Based on the assumption that psychological problems often stem from erroneous patterns of thinking and distorted perceptions of reality, cognitive interventions try to establish new belief systems that enable the patient to reinterpret and reintegrate her/his experiences (e.g., Beck, Rush, Shaw, & Emery, 1979). *Socratic dialogue, cognitive restructuring, or paradoxical intervention* are techniques used to identify and modify dysfunctional perceptions and beliefs.

Desensitization and exposure techniques try to improve coping and tolerance of the stressor (*in sensu* or *in vivo*; e.g., Stampfl & Lewis, 1967), especially when there is anxiety involved. They aim at reducing the arousal caused by the stressor through repeated confrontation and habituation (Wolpe, 1958, EMDR, Shapiro, 1989). The patient is confronted with the feared stimuli in a step by step manner while she/he is relaxed, distracted or eliciting trained positive cognitions or emotions, until she/he is able to tolerate the adverse stimuli.

Training of coping strategies, such as assertiveness training (e.g., Ullrich de Muynck & Ullrich, 1976), aim at improving skills required of the patient so that he or she can better master the stressor or in a more general way promote self-efficacy (e.g., Bandura, 1977).

Contextual-ecological interventions are based on the assumption that the dysfunction is not only a function of the individual, but also of the social context in which the individual is entrenched. The psychotherapeutic techniques used in this context intend to build up positive social activities (e.g., Brown & Munford, 1984) in order to prevent social reclusion and isolation. In order to achieve this, variables from different contexts, such as work, family, peer group, or leisure time, are analyzed and worked on.

Only few data are available on pharmacological treatment. Benzodiazepines are used, especially for patients with severe life stress and a significant anxiety component. For patients with current or past substance abuse, tricyclic antidepressants or buspirone have been recommended (Strain et al. 1999). There are almost no controlled clinical trials in this field and no drug which is specifically marketed for adjustment disorders.

Since PTSD was included as a separate psychological disorder in the DSM in 1980 (APA, 1980), a growing number of scientific intervention studies have emerged on this special form of reactive disorder. A review of 29 studies (Blake & Sonnenberg, 1998) showed that cognitive therapy reduced symptoms like sleep disturbance, intrusions, depersonalization, depression, dysfunctional cognitions, avoidance behavior, and numbing. Behavioral interventions proved to be effective in reducing anxiety-related symptoms of PTSD like hyperarousal, increased heart frequency, fear experience, and intrusions.

Adjustment disorders in clinical practice

Even though there is scientific evidence that adjustment disorders are frequent conditions, especially in primary care, adjustment disorders do not seem to be diagnosed very often. Their diagnostic status has always been controversial (Casey et al. 2001). Fard, Hudgens, & Welner, (1979) speak of a "wastebasket diagnosis, used in such a vague and all encompassing manner as to be useless." The diagnostic criteria are so vague that such a diagnosis cannot tell anything about the present clinical problem (Andreasen, & Wasek, 1980; Fabrega et al. 1987; Snyder et al. 1990; Bronisch, & Hecht, 1989; Bronisch, 1991; Pollock, 1992; Despland, Monod, & Ferrero, 1995; Greenberg, Rosenfeld, & Ortega, 1995; Jones, Yates, Williams, Zhou, & Hardman, 1999; Casey et al. 2001; Linden, 2003). It is poorly defined, overlaps with other diagnostic groupings, presents problems of reliability and validity, and has an undefined symptomatology.

Strain et al. (1999), on the other hand, have argued that because of its imprecision, the diagnostic category of adjustment disorders is useful in psychiatry. Emerging illnesses are difficult to identify in early stages, and in such instances the diagnosis of adjustment disorders can serve as a temporary diagnosis that can be modified with information from longitudinal evaluation and treatment. From this point of view, the diagnosis of adjustment disorders appears as a way of "tagging" an individual for possible difficulty before the morbidity becomes apparent. Thus, the diagnosis of adjustment disorders serves as a transient, subthreshold diagnosis, which lies in the gray area between normal behavior and mental disorders.

There is also some scientific evidence to support that adjustment disorders are a valid diagnosis (Despland et al. 1995). A comparison between subjects with adjustment disorders, with specific disorders, and without mental problems resulted in the conclusion that subjects with adjustment disorders differ from the other two groups in respect to severity of symptoms, psychosocial adaptation, and number and intensity of stressors (Fabrega et al. 1987).

A reason why adjustment disorders are subject to such controversial discussion could well be that these patients are not seen in traditional psychiatric settings and therefore do not get the necessary scientific attention. There have been fewer than 30 publications in peer-reviewed journals over the past 25 years exclusively devoted to adjustment disorders (Casey et al. 2001).

An important reason for giving more attention to the group of adjustment disorders is that both in clinical practice and in the scientific literature the diagnostic of PTSD is used in an ever more pervasive manner. Reactions to life events which are not life threatening and fear provoking but still cause persistent psychological changes are given a diagnosis of PTSD (Linden, Schippan, Baumann & Spielberg, 2004). This threatens the specificity of the PTSD diagnosis and indicates the necessity to further subclassify adjustment disorders. Given this background and modeled on PTSD, Linden (2003) described Posttraumatic Embitterment Disorder (PTED) as a distinct subgroup of adjustment disorders in which the trigger event is not an anxiety-provoking and life-threatening stimulus but an exceptional, though normal negative life event.

1.3 Posttraumatic Embitterment Disorder (PTED)

The clinical problem

It is know that burdensome societal events, like war or natural disaster, which affect many people at a time can be accompanied by an increase in the prevalence of reactive disorders such as PTSD. The German reunification of 1990 forced 17 million people in the former German Democratic Republic (GDR) to reorganize their lives, and in many cases this had to happen several times during the following years. Many biographies made unexpected turns because of changes in the economic, legal, and cultural system. Individuals who thought that they could foresee their career suddenly had to realize that their qualifications were no longer honored. Public servants in high positions suddenly had to sell insurance contracts or drive a taxi. Individuals who had previously enjoyed a high rank in society lost their status. And furthermore, there was a general feeling that East Germans were second-class citizens. In a public survey in 2002, 59% of those interviewed said that there were still big differences between East and West, and only 1% thought that the two parts were fully integrated. Only 20% felt they were "full citizens of the Federal Republic of Germany." 30% had experienced a biographical downgrading and 10% wanted the GDR to be reinstated (Winkler 2002). In some areas, more than 50% of voters voted for the socialist party that succeeded the former communist party as late as the 2005 elections.

Within the same period, a growing number of individuals suffering from severe and prolonged deterioration of their overall mental status sought treatment. The onset of problems was regularly related to a specific event of frustration, downgrading, or humiliation. In respect to onset, course, and symptoms they did not fit into any diagnostic categories of DSM-IV and ICD-10. As the leading psychopathological characteristic was persistent and nagging embitterment, this disorder was described as "Posttraumatic Embitterment Disorder (PTED)" (Linden, 2003) and conceptualized as a special form of adjustment disorder with its own etiology and psychopathological characteristics. This type of reaction is not specific to a special event like the German reunification but also occurs in many other patients and circumstances. The trigger event in PTED is an exceptional, though normal negative life event such as conflict in the workplace, unemployment, the death of a relative, divorce, severe illness, or experience of loss or separation. The illness develops in the direct context of the event. Characteristic is a prolonged feeling of embitterment. Additional symptoms are intrusive thoughts and avoidance of situations or objects which are connected to the event, self-blame, anger, depression, hopelessness, phobia, somatic symptoms, or suicidal tendencies. As a consequence, performance in daily activities is impaired. In the following, a case vignette will be presented, followed by a detailed outline of the emotion embitterment and a description of research diagnostic criteria together with theories on the psychological background.

Case vignette

A 55-year-old man lost his job because of a reorganization of the children's home in which he had worked for many years. He did not show any sign of mental disorder before this critical life event but was a rather tolerant and efficient person who was well accepted by the children and by colleagues. In the immediate context of the negative life event, the patient started to develop a persistent disorder with a chronic and deteriorating course with disabling consequences. Symptoms were negative mood, self-directed blame, hopelessness, and multiple unspecific somatic complaints such as sleep disturbance and loss of appetite. The clinical picture somewhat resembled melancholic depression (Rush & Weissenburger 1995). He also developed phobic behavior and tried to avoid places and persons which would remind him of his former work or confront him with former colleagues or even people who could possibly know about his misfortune. These phobic reactions had a clear tendency to be triggered by ever more distant, less relevant stimuli, resembling agoraphobia. In contrast to depression, he experienced event-related aggression and no impairment in modulation of mood. If he was reminded of the critical event, he reacted with emotional outbursts. If he was made to imagine some kind of revenge on "the western system" or his old employer, the patient smiled and underwent a complete change in emotional status. Such vengeful thoughts were that the children's home would go bankrupt or even that the unified Germany would loose its economic power. As opposed to findings in depression, fully normal affect could be observed when he was occupied with some distracting activity. The patient was on prolonged sick leave and his marriage was endangered because his status was a severe burden on his wife and because he refused to participate in any social activities.

The explanation for this impressive reaction was the matching nature of personal history and belief systems on the one hand and the type of critical event on the other. The patient had been a social worker in a church-owned children's home. He had therefore always been somewhat distant from the old political system. When reunification came, he full-heartedly looked forward to

Table 1. Case vignette of PTED

---

1. Life event
Male, 55 years. Lost his job as a social worker because of a reorganization of the institution in which he had worked for many years.

2. Premorbid personality and functioning
The patient worked as social worker in a children's home for many
years. He was well accepted by the children and by his colleagues. He
personally saw to it that the children's home survived during the organi-
zational turmoil in the first years after German reunification and prevented closure of the home.

3. Subjective interpretation of the event
For years he had been a man who put enormous effort into his job as a
social worker. As a member of the church, he had always been in some
opposition to the old socialist system. He had expected a lot from the
political changes. However, it was the new system and especially the
church that - for him, unexpectedly and unjustly - made him redundant.

4. Emotional reaction
Mention of his work resulted in immediate outbursts of dysphoric and
aggressive emotions, strong vegetative reactions, and high tension. He
broke out in tears and clenched his fists. For moments he could be totally absent-minded and in a dissociative state. He called himself a failure,
someone who could not even feed his family, a cripple who should best
be killed. He suffered from severe sleep disorders, loss of libido, lack of
drive, and neglect of his appearance. He showed phobic symptoms such
as avoidance of all situations and places where he possibly could meet
his former colleagues. He showed suicidal ideation and rejected help.

5. Modulation of affect
When distracted, he showed unimpaired emotions and was even able to
laugh. When thoughts of revenge against the "system," the church, or
the new managers were stimulated. he started to grin all over his face.

6. Duration
Fifteen months until now

7. Social consequences
The patient declined new job offers, did not look after his personal af-
fairs, and withdrew from his family and friends

better times. In the turmoil of those days he almost personally made sure that the children's home was not closed. He identified himself very much with the work he did. The children's home was then taken over by a "western" church affiliation. They now reorganized the home and dismissed several employees. As he was one of the older workers, he was the first to be sacked, while younger and less experienced colleagues stayed in their jobs. This came as a complete surprise to him, as he had expected that his special services would be valued. In the light of many years of good service and in view of his personal system of values, he experienced this as unjust, hurtful, a degradation and a devaluation of what he had built up over the years. The emotional consequence was embitterment. The main characteristics of this case vignette are summarized in Table 1.

Embitterment

Embitterment is, of course, not a new human experience. In ancient times, it was described as follows by Aristotle (Susemihl, 1912): "Embittered are those who cannot be reconciled, who keep their rancor, they hold their arousal in themselves, not coming to rest unless revenge has come. Revenge reduces arousal and changes pain into contentment. Does this not happen, then the pressure grows. As the internal turmoil does not open itself to others, nobody can counsel and help. It needs time to overcome internal arousal. Those persons are a burden to themselves and their dearest friends."

Today, bitterness and embitterment are terms that are frequently used in colloquial discourse. They are used in politics, culture, sport, and economics.[7] Various "embittered" characters can also be encountered in literature. A prime example is the scientist Victor Frankenstein in Mary Shelley's novel "Frankenstein" (1818). Victor Frankenstein is an idealist who believes in scientific progress. In his scientific eagerness, he creates an artificial human being. However, when he becomes aware of the ugliness and wretchedness of his creation, he abandons it. When the creation turns against his friends and relatives, Frankenstein realizes with bitterness that his desire to be useful to the human race has led him to create a threat to humankind. All his dreams and values are shattered. He reacts with despair, melancholy, and sorrow. The man who had been driven by the belief in scientific progress and usefulness loses all he had hoped for in the face of his creation. In the following, he remains unable to take responsibility for what he has done. And only after his creation has destroyed his life by killing his relatives and friends, is Frankenstein able to find a new motive in his life, revenge. However, this motive only drives him to

---

[7] For a detailed description of the use of the term "embitterment" in the media, see Albrecht (2004).

chase after something he can never reach. Finally, in his struggle for revenge, Frankenstein dies of exhaustion.

The dictionary of contemporary English (Langenscheid-Longman, 1995) defines the term "to embitter" as "to make someone feel hate and anger for a long time because they think they have been treated unfairly." To feel embittered therefore describes a prolonged emotional state of hate and anger caused by the belief that one has been treated unfairly. In the German Duden dictionary of word meanings (Duden, 1985; p. 696), embitterment is defined as: "to bear a grudge against one's own fate, which is experienced as too harsh, or against a treatment that is experienced as injust." The online version of the classic German dictionary compiled by Jacob and Wilhelm Grimm (2005) defines embitterment as a personal trait or prolonged condition, while the term bitterness describes a transient emotional arousal. The "eLook online dictionary" (2005) lists the terms envenom and acerbate as synonyms for embitter.

Due to the frequent use of bitterness and embitterment, the understanding of these terms is not confined to their definitions, and many different meanings can be encountered in colloquial language. Here, emotions, cognitions, and attitudes as well as certain behaviors are all aspects of embitterment. Schaad (2002) defined embitterment as an "emotion-guided behavior complex." He tried to categorize different meanings of embitterment that can be found in colloquial language and identified four different groups:

- self-consciousness, fear, anxiety, mistrust
- despair, contempt, displeasure, anger, rage, fury, antipathy, indignation, hate, hostility, malevolence, aggressiveness, derision, displeasure, revenge, disdain, arrogance, stinginess, envy, toughness, sadism, rigidity
- grief, melancholy, sorrow, oppression, depression, aloofness, misery, pessimism, aversion, weariness, hopelessness, boredom, dissatisfaction, disappointment, indifference
- obsessiveness, stubbornness, individualism, dogmatism, fanaticism.

Only a few scientific studies have addressed the emotion embitterment. Pirhacova (1997) described embitterment as caused by social injustice. Zemperl and Frese (1997) observed this emotion as a reaction to protracted unemployment. Baures (1996) mentioned embitterment and hate in connection with extreme trauma, and emphasized the importance of letting go of these destructive emotions, in order to recover. Webster (1993) addressed bitterness revival as a function of reminiscence. Znoj (2002) developed an "embitterment scale" when working with cancer patients. Alexander (1966) made an attempt to study the phenomenology of bitterness in psychoanalytical terms. In his view, the feeling of bitterness is a universal experience that does not constitute a clinical or sociological problem unless the affect is quantitatively great. Even though bitterness is often encountered in a clinical context, the affect is usually not experienced as morbid. It is rather seen as an unpleasant feeling justified by external reality, hence appropriate, and therefore not a sickness. Patients therefore tend to go in the direction of making demands for the redress of the grievances, and do not seek treatment.

So far, the term embitterment has not been introduced into the psychological and psychiatric nomenclature. No entries can be found in prominent psychological dictionaries (Colman, 2003; Häcker & Stapf, 1998). While, for example, the index of the *Textbook of Psychiatry* (Hales et al. 1999) shows 42 references related to anxiety and 53 references related to depression, no reference to embitterment can be found. In addition, embitterment is not listed in psychopathological systems like the AMDP-system (AMDP, 1995) or the list of technical terms in DSM-IV (APA, 1994).

Embitterment is a distinct state of mood. It differs from depression, hopelessness, and also anger as such, though it can share common emotional features or exist in parallel with each of these other emotions. In contrast to anger, it has the additional quality of self-blame and a feeling of injustice. One can be angry at somebody without being embittered. Embitterment is an emotion of having been let down, a feeling and cognition of injustice together with the drive to fight back but not being able to find one's proper goal. Embitterment is nagging and self-increasing. It does not end by itself but goes on and on. Embittered individuals recall the insulting event over and over again. This is similar to intrusive thoughts in PTSD (McFarlane, 1992). The difference is that, in embitterment, emotions sometimes seem to be hurting and rewarding at the same time. There is even something addictive to memories of the trigger events. This could also be because embittered individuals feel the need to persuade others of the strength of their cause. There are also feelings of revenge. Individuals who suffer from embitterment can, in the blink of an eye, turn from terrifying despair to smiles at the thought that revenge could be theirs. These characteristic features of embitterment illustrate the vast pathological properties of this emotion.

With PTED, Linden (2003) introduced a concept that for the first time thoroughly acknowledges the emotion embitterment and its possible pathological consequences. In PTED, embitterment develops in the aftermath of a negative life event. It encompasses persistent feelings of being let down, insulted, or having lost, and of being revengeful but helpless.

Research diagnostic criteria for PTED

Based on theoretical considerations and clinical experience, Linden (2003) introduced research diagnostic criteria for PTED (see Table 2). Necessary for

Table 2. Research diagnostic criteria for PTED

A. Core criteria

1. A single exceptional negative life event precipitates the onset of the illness.
2. Patients know about this life event and see their present negative state as a direct and lasting consequence of this event.
3. Patients experience the negative life event as "unjust" and respond with embitterment and emotional arousal when reminded of the event.
4. No obvious mental disorder in the year before the critical event. The present state is no recurrence of a preexisting mental disorder.

B. Additional signs and symptoms

1. Patients see themselves as victims and as helpless/unable to cope with the event or the cause.
2. Patients blame themselves for the event, for not having prevented it, or for not being able to cope with it.
3. Patients report repeated intrusive memories of the critical event. They partly even think that it is important not to forget.
4. Patients express thoughts that it does no longer matter how they are doing and are even uncertain whether they want the wounds to heal.
5. Patients can express suicidal ideation.
6. Additional emotions are dysphoria, aggression, down-heartedness, which can resemble melancholic depressive states with somatic syndromes.
6. Patients show a variety of unspecific somatic complaints such as loss of appetite, sleep disturbance, pain.
7. Patients can report phobic symptoms in respect to the place or to persons related to the event.
8. Drive is reduced and blocked. Patients experience themselves not so much as drive inhibited but rather as drive unwilling.
9. Emotional modulation is not impaired and patients can show normal affect when they are distracted or even smile when engaged in thoughts of revenge.

C. Duration: Symptoms last for longer than 3 months.

D. Impairment: Performance in daily activities and roles is impaired.

---

the diagnosis of PTED is a critical event that is a normal but not everyday event, and that is in this respect exceptional. The patients see it as the cause of their present state and of a persistent negative change in their well-being. The patient perceives the event as injust and has the feeling that she or he is a victim. When reminded of the event, typical emotional reactions, especially embitterment, can be observed. Characteristic symptoms, similar to PTSD, are intrusive thoughts (McFarlane, 1992) and repetitive memories of the event, eliciting accompanying negative emotions. Affect modulation is unimpaired and normal affect can be observed if the patient is distracted.

This reaction cannot be explained by some mental disorder, psychopathology, maladaptation, or impaired functioning prior to the event and the symptoms cannot be attributed to any other psychiatric disorder. This can be a difficult diagnostic problem especially in regard to personality disorders. In the psychiatric tradition there are numerous terms which refer in one way or the other to personalities which fight and bite without asking for the outcome, and where there are psychopathological exacerbations when life problems occur. Examples are *querulous paranoia*, *paranoid personality*, *passive-aggressive personality*, or *hostile depression*. Furthermore, there is the problem that individuals who react to a special event with PTED may have experienced similar events and earlier trauma before, which function as "feeder memories." These diagnostic problems cannot be solved entirely nor answered in all cases with a yes or a no. They are similarly known from PTSD (McKenzie, Marks, & Liness, 2001). Therefore, the diagnostic approach should be pragmatic. There should be no obvious premorbid psychopathology or functional disorder before the critical event and there should be a clear change in this respect after the event.

The core signs and symptoms of PTED can be accompanied by self-blame, anger, depression, hopelessness, phobia, or somatic symptoms. The duration of the disorder is longer than three months and daily role performance is impaired.

The spectrum of critical events

As shown in the case vignette, PTED develops in the immediate context of a negative life event. Patients who did not show any sign of mental disorder previous to the event develop impressive psychopathological symptoms in the aftermath of a single negative event. The common feature of such events is that they are experienced as unjust, as a personal insult, and psychologically as a violation of basic beliefs and values (Beck et al. 1979).

Events that can lead to embitterment can happen in every life domain. In a study by Linden et al. (2004), the trigger event was work related in 62% of cases, related to the family or partnership in 14%, in 14% it was the death of a relative or a friend, and in 10% something else.

The posttraumatic nature of the illness

Smith, Bem & Nolen-Hoeksema (2001) define traumatic events as situations of objective extreme danger that are outside the range of usual human experience. These include natural disasters, such as earthquakes and floods; manmade disasters such as wars and nuclear accidents; catastrophic accidents, such as car or plane crashes; and physical assaults, such as rape or attempted murder. In this respect, PTSD is rightfully called a "posttraumatic" disorder.

Given this definition, one could ask if the term "trauma" is also appropriate in PTED. The trigger events in PTED are exceptional but usual life events that do not encompass extreme danger, or a threat to one's physical integrity. There are, however, four reasons to use the term posttraumatic also in PTED.

Firstly, as already discussed before, psychological research has shown that the meaning of an event for a particular individual cannot be defined by objective characteristics (e.g., extreme danger), but by the individual's personal perception of the event. This is even true for "danger" or "life-threatening events". By integrating the subjective meaning of an event, a patient-centered definition of "trauma" is put forward. This definition of trauma follows the view that the individual interpretation of a stressor must be taken into account in order to determine the amount of stress experienced (e.g., Schwarzer & Schulz, 2002; Filipp, 1995; Lazarus 1966). We assume that the violation of basic beliefs in PTED is experienced as "traumatic" by the individual concerned. The pathogenic mechanism in PTED is not an event-inherent property, but emerges from the match between the belief and value system of the patient on one side, and the violation of these beliefs by the event on the other. This threat to deeply-held beliefs acts as a powerful psychological shock upon the patient.

Secondly, the critical events are also "threatening" in nature. Although they may not be "life threatening," they will nevertheless affect every individual in a negative way. The loss of a job or public humiliation is negative and burdensome for almost everyone. In any case it will put a strain on the individual and provoke an adaptive response.

Thirdly, there is a psychopathological response which is by and large specific to traumatic experiences. Intrusive thoughts and repetitive memories of the event, eliciting accompanying negative emotions, characterize both PTSD and PTED. Moreover, many PTED patients also report phobic symptoms in respect to places or persons related to the event.

Fourthly, there is the course of time. There are patients who fall from full health to a state of total despair, helplessness, downheartedness and embitterment from one second to the next. This "causal" relationship is so evident that there is no better term but "posttraumatic".

Differential diagnosis

Despite overlaps in symptomatology, PTED is a separate form of adjustment disorder (ICD-10, F 43.2; DSM-IV, 309). The essential feature of adjustment disorder is the development of clinically relevant emotional or behavioral symptoms in response to an identifiable psychosocial stressor. This is true for PTED, in which a negative life event precipitates the onset of the illness. Thus, PTED and adjustment disorder are both diagnoses with a known etiology, in which the etiological agent is central to the diagnosis. While the diagnosis of adjustment disorder offers no criteria to qualify and quantify stressors or to assess their effect or meaning for a particular individual at a given time, in PTED, the stressor is defined as an event which is experienced as unjust, as a personal insult, and psychologically as a violation of basic beliefs and values. The examples of stressors given in ICD-10 and DSM-IV (e.g., termination of a romantic relationship, marked business difficulties) that may cause adjustment disorder can occur in PTED. But here, it is not the content or type but rather the humiliating or frustrating nature of the event that's important. In addition, adjustment disorders are understood as limited in time and should show remission after some months (see Chapter 1.2.). In contrast to this, the symptomatology found in PTED does not show a tendency towards spontaneous remission.

Given its chronic course, PTED could possibly be allocated to the class of enduring personality change after catastrophic experience (ICD-10, F 62.0). However, this would miss the specificity of the emotional reaction, i.e., embitterment. This is a very distinct state of mind which can and should be kept separate from other negative "personality traits," such as general hostile and distrustful attitudes towards the world or interactional difficulties.

In some patients, PTED can at first glance be similar to depression and in some cases even resemble melancholic depression, due to persistent negative mood and inhibition of drive. However, in contrast to depression, there is no impairment of modulation of affect. PTED patients can show normal mood when distracted or engaged in revenge fantasies. Furthermore, the diagnosis of depression does not catch the full spectrum of emotions. Persistent rancor and thoughts of revenge are not symptoms of depression. Also, intrusive memories and emotional outbursts in reaction to being reminded of the critical event are not typical for depression. Although negative life events in the patient's history are also often found in depression, depressive patients do not react as PTED patients do. Usually there is some form of continuous strain rather than an acute and specific event.

When contrasting PTED with PTSD, important differences are the type of critical event experienced and the type of emotional reaction. In PTSD, there must be an exceptional, life-threatening event which provokes panic and anxiety. In PTED, there is an event that can be called normal as it can happen to many people in a life course, such as divorce or redundancy and unemployment. Still, it is also an exceptional event in that it is not an everyday event for an individual. While in PTSD anxiety is the predominant emotion, in PTED it is embitterment.

PTED can also show overlaps with anxiety disorders such as agoraphobia. Some patients show clear avoidance behavior. They do not leave the house or go shopping. In contrast to agoraphobia, there is a clear relation of this behavior to the critical event in individuals suffering from PTED. They do not pass by their former workplace as they do not want to be reminded of what happened and to endure the resulting negative and hurting emotions. They do not go out in public as they do not want to encounter anyone who knows about their misery.

1.4 Basic Beliefs and PTED

Explanations for reactions to life events

The question why some individuals show such an impressive reaction to a negative life event that, although severe, is not outside the range of normal life events, can at present only be answered speculatively with reference to clinical impression and early research.

Every life event interacts with psychological and biological factors, personal history or situational factors. General dimensions of interest could be alexithymia, irritable mood, demoralization, or denial. Situational and event-related dimensions of interest are, for example, the sense of threat, or the type and extent of loss or change in living conditions (Madianos, Papaghelis, Ioannovich, & Dafni, 2001; Kjaer Fuglsang, Moergeli, Hepp-Beg, & Schnyder, 2002). Finally, resilience must be taken into account, factors such as sense of coherence, perceived invulnerability, coping repertoire, or preparedness for a traumatic experience (Timko, & Janoff-Bulman, 1985; Basoglu, Mineka, Paker, Aker, Livanou, & Gok, 1997; Staudinger, Freund, Linden, & Maas, 1999; Schnyder, Buchi, Sensky, & Klaghofer, 2000).

Interesting avenues in the explanation of why embitterment develops can be found in cognitive theories. There is the concept of self-blame, be it behavioral or characterological (Janoff-Bulman, 1979), although it is difficult to say whether this is an antecedent or a consequence of trauma (Frazier, 1990; Shaver, & Drown, 1986; Livanou, Basoglu, Marks, De, Noshirvani, Lovell, & Thrasher, 2002). The same is true for general assumptions about the meaning and benevolence of the world (Magwaza, 1999).

Another interesting question is the role of revenge or compensation, and whether embitterment would be prevented if this was possible. PTED patients often complain that there has been no justice. However, if there is justice this is typically never enough. As revenge is out of reach, at least in the perception of those who seek treatment as patients, aggression can be turned against the self and self-blame can become a prominent psychopathological feature (Janoff-Bulman, 1979). Patients can blame themselves for not having been competent enough to avoid the event or for not having done things that could have prevented the disaster. Some almost love to degrade themselves and even reject offers of help and compensation. They prefer the world to see how badly they have been treated. For the patient described in the case vignette above, we arranged for a new job to be offered to him elsewhere, which he refused to accept, as this would have meant to just "forget" what had been done to him.

This underlying aggression can be a major problem in treating these patients, as it can also turn against the therapist.

Violation of basic beliefs

PTED is a reactive disorder triggered by an exceptional, though normal negative life event, such as conflict in the workplace, unemployment, death of a relative, or divorce. One common characteristic of such events, according to concepts of cognitive psychotherapy, is a violation of basic beliefs and values (Beck et al. 1979; Janoff-Bulman, 1992; Basoglu et al. 1997; see also above).

An example would be a woman for whom the family is the most important thing in life, who has sacrificed her career to support her husband and to take care of the children, and who, years later, is left by her husband for a younger woman. Most importantly, the children choose to live with their father. As a result, the personal value system of the woman is called into question. The basic belief in the value and worth of a "good" family life, which gave her live structure and meaning, suddenly crumbles. The question is whether she has "wasted" her life and put everything on the wrong card. Somthing similar could happen if an individual gets sacked, even though they have shown great commitment and dedication in their job. These examples demonstrate that personal value systems that make people successful in certain life domains are at the same time a vulnerability factor (Schippan et al. 2004).

In regard to premorbid personality, patients with PTED seem to be achievement oriented, devoted persons with strict convictions and beliefs. They often showed great self-sacrifice and commitment in their job or social role before the critical event. Given this background, negative events like redundancy, divorce, or mobbing are experienced as a major insult, abasement and humiliation. Central assumptions of self-worth, of a just and benevolent world are violated. Even though the event does not threaten the individual's physical integrity, it is nevertheless experienced as traumatic, as it threatens the veracity of their fundamental assumptions and the associated emotions.

Basic beliefs have been described in different theoretical contexts. Bolby (1969) referred to "internal world models," Marris (1975) to "structures of meaning," Kelly (1955) to "personal constructs," Parkes (1975) and Janoff-Bulman (1985; 1990; Janoff-Bulman & Frieze, 1983) to "assumptive worlds," and Epstein (1973) to "personal theories of reality." Additionally, researchers studying the psychological aftermath of trauma (Collins, Taylor, & Skokan, 1990; Epstein, 1980; Janoff-Bulman & Frieze, 1983; Schwartzberg & Janoff-Bulman, 1991; Taylor, 1983) have focused their attention on changes in people's basic beliefs about themselves and the world. They have proposed that stressors affect adjustment in part because they challenge people's basic beliefs about themselves and the world.

The term "basic beliefs" refers to a cognitive framework that structures experience and influences perception and behavior, enabling people to experience the world as predictable and controllable (Rini, Manne, DuHamel, Austin, Ostroff, Boulad, Parsons, Marini, Williams, Mee, Sexon, & Redd, 2004). These basic beliefs lie at the core of our inner world and generally go unquestioned and unchallenged (Bowlby, 1969; Epstein, 1973; Parkes, 1975). Basic beliefs are learned in childhood and adolescence and comprise abstract beliefs about ourselves, the external world, and the relationship between the two. Through early social interactions, we develop a view of the world and ourselves that enables us to develop a "sense of basic trust" towards the world and ourselves (Erikson, 1968).

Janoff-Bulman (1992) distinguished three major basic beliefs: a) people tend to believe in the benevolence of people and the world; b) they tend to believe that people usually get what they deserve and that positive and negative outcome can be controlled by engaging in appropriate behavior; c) they tend to hold positive self-beliefs. Based on these assumptions the world is perceived as a nonrandom, meaningful place. People believe that outcomes are not randomly distributed; rather, there is a relation between an individual and what happens to him or her, a person-outcome contingency that "makes sense." Hence, negative events happen to certain people because of who they are (e.g., immoral attributes) or what they do (e.g., careless action). This assumption of meaningfulness, of a predictive, nonrandom world, enables people to feel safe and secure. It allows to maintain an illusion of relative invulnerability (Janoff-Bulman, 1998). The three positive assumptions about the world coexist at the core of our assumptive world. They are not narrow beliefs, but broad, abstract conceptions that are emotionally potent. It feels good to believe that we are decent and the world is benevolent and meaningful. Thus, positive feelings are inextricably tied to our fundamental assumptions (Janoff-Bulman, 1992).

According to Janoff-Bulman (1989), traumatic events may shatter fundamental assumptions and beliefs about the world. The new information on the experience of trauma may no longer match the old assumptions. Because traumatic events are too vivid and powerful to discount, the major task confronting victims of trauma is to assimilate new trauma data into their basic beliefs, to rework the data to fit their old assumptions, or to adjust their basic beliefs about themselves and the world to accommodate the new information (Magwaza, 1999). If the veracity of basic beliefs is challenged by a stressor, adjustment to such an event is influenced by an individual's ability to rebuild and adjust basic beliefs in light of it (Creamer, Burgess, & Pattison, 1992; Janoff-Bulman, 1992; Taylor, 1983).

Guided by the hypothesis that PTSD is caused by a disconfirmation of the basic beliefs in a personal theory of reality (Epstein, 1991), Fletcher (1988, summarized in Epstein, 1991) examined the influence of an extremely stressful life event (combat) on basic beliefs in Vietnam war veterans. The magnitude of change in basic beliefs was most profound in veterans with symptoms of PTSD as compared to veterans without symptoms of PTSD, and a noncombat group. Moreover, whereas the other groups exhibited marked recovery in the favorability of their basic beliefs several months after discharge, the favorability of the basic beliefs of the PTSD group continued to decline until the last period rated, which, for most, was more than 15 years after their combat experience.

The shattering of basic beliefs in the aftermath of trauma such as combat experiences, rape, or natural disasters represents an exceptional, extreme act. In the normal course of events, the instance of change in our fundamental assumptions is rare. Our basic beliefs serve as guides that enable us to make sense of our world, to understand and integrate events in our world. They guide coherent behavior over the life cycle of an individual, and even over generations of groups and whole nations. This makes them resistant to change, even when confronted with opposing evidence (Linden, 2003). Cognitively, we are conservative. We tend to maintain our theories about us and the world rather than change them; we interpret information so as to be schema-consistent, we behave in ways that serve to confirm our preexisting beliefs, and we discount or isolate contradictory evidence so that our preexisting schemas remain intact (Janoff-Bulman, 1992). Within the field of clinical psychology, Beck and colleagues (Beck et al. 1979) emphasized the importance of schema-consistent biases. They suggested that negative schemas are involved in the distortion and inaccuracies associated with all types of psychopathology.

Similar to PTSD, the impressive reaction evident in PTED can be explained in terms of a disconfirmation of basic beliefs and values caused by the negative life event. However, the negative life event in PTED does not shatter fundamental assumptions; rather, the event stands for a violation of basic beliefs and values. Thus, basic beliefs remain intact in PTED. In PTSD, the traumatic event shatters the basic assumptions (e.g., belief in relative invulnerability) that provide psychological coherence and stability in a complex world. Hence, the predominant emotional experience of trauma victims is intense fear and anxiety (Janoff-Bulman, 1992). In PTED, the predominant emotion is embitterment, which results from the contradiction between core beliefs and the negative event. Patients with PTED hold on to their fundamental assumptions. They maintain their core beliefs and go on to interpret the world in light of them. It is this strict adherence to their basic beliefs that can explain the prolonged emotional reaction to the trigger event. The negative event represents a constant threat to fundamental assumptions, and at the same time it is too vivid and powerful to discount.

In the literature on PTSD and negative life events (Schützwohl, & Maercker, 2000; Ehlers, Clark, Dunmore, Jaycox, Meadows, & Foa, 1998; Ehlers, Maercker, & Boos, 2000), it is proposed that one important dimension of trauma is that one's personal integrity has been threatened. The concept proposed here is close to these observations but it goes one step further. We regard not only the threat to personal integrity as a key feature of the disorder but any violation of basic beliefs.

The model of a violation of basic beliefs in PTED can explain why the prevalence of this disorder must increase in times of social change. Just as a higher rate of PTSD can be observed in times of war or in populations exposed to major catastrophies that threaten the life of many people (Kulka et al. 1990), social changes (and the German reunification is a good example) can be expected to increase the risk of PTED.

During the nineties, most East Germans underwent enormous changes in their biographies, almost everybody had to cope with fundamental changes in their work situation and in their families, and many saw their value systems called into question. Even those who seem to be better off today than before live under greater uncertainty in respect to their individual future as compared to their lives under the socialist regime (Hillen, Schaub, Hiestermann, Kirchner, & Robra, 2000). There are men and women who feel that much of their life has been wasted because of the old system and even those who hoped for a new beginning in the new system often found that they were cheated, let down, or set aside. It is because of these large social changes that we have seen more cases of PTED, and that the similarities and features of this disorder have become obvious. However, PTED can also occur in other contexts.

It is likely that there is a base rate of PTED in normal times as well, since humiliation or injustice are as frequent a life experience as car accidents or life-threatening events, leading to enduring negative consequences of clinical relevance in at least some people. We assume that PTED can be seen at all times in all places.

1.5 Wisdom and PTED

Wisdom Psychology

Wisdom and basic beliefs

The question is how an individual can adjust to violations of basic beliefs. An inherent psychological problem is that basic beliefs are very resistant to change even when confronted with disconfirming information. The inflexibility of basic beliefs as found in PTED can best be described by referring to modern wisdom psychology (Erikson, 1976; Baltes & Smith, 1990; Staudinger & Baltes, 1996a; Staudinger, Lopez, Baltes, 1997). Wisdom has been defined as "expert knowledge in the fundamental pragmatics of life" (Baltes & Staudinger, 2000) and as a knowledge system that enables a person to deal with complex and difficult life problems. This ability is particularly required when an individual is confronted with negative life events that threaten basic beliefs and values. In this vein, wisdom-related problem solving strategies can be seen as contrary to rigid, dogmatic, one-sided, emotion-guided, and inflexible thinking that facilitates embitterment and self-destructive resignation. Wisdom as knowledge about fundamental aspects of life such as chance, uncertainty, and our own fragility appears to put our basic beliefs into perspective, and facilitates adjustment if our core beliefs fail to match reality.

In this regard, it is hypothesized that a deficiency in activating wisdom strategies when confronted with difficult life problems can foster the development of PTED. This chapter describes the field of wisdom research and introduces a conceptualization of wisdom for the clinical context.

History of psychological research on wisdom

For millennia, wisdom has been considered an ideal and pinnacle of human development (e.g., Assman, 1994; Baltes, 1995; Baltes & Smith, 1990; Robinson, 1990; Staudinger & Baltes, 1994). It is an ideal for which individuals strive, which regulates the direction of development but which is very difficult to achieve (Staudinger & Baltes, 1996b). Wisdom is thought to be an integrative link between mind and virtue (Baltes & Staudinger, 2000). Wise people are thought to possess many positive qualities, such as a mature and integrated personality, superior judgment skills in difficult life matters, and the ability to cope with the vicissitudes of life (Assmann, 1994; Ardelt, 2004; Bianchi, 1994; Clayton, 1982; Dittman-Kohli & Baltes, 1990; Kekes, 1983, 1995; Kramer, 2000; Sternberg, 1990, 1998; Vaillant, 1993).

During the last two decades, researchers in the behavioral sciences have shown renewed interest in the ancient concept of wisdom (Chinen, 1984; Clayton & Birren, 1980; Dittman-Kohli & Baltes, Sternberg, 1990). A possible reason for this resurrection is a new emphasis on positive psychology (Ardelt, 2004). However, because of the culturally rich meaning and heritage of wisdom, defining and operationalizing the concept of wisdom as a scientifically grounded psychological construct is not easy (Baltes & Staudinger, 2000). Hall (1922) was one of the first psychologists to tackle this task. Subsequently, it was primarily the lifespan model of Erikson (1976) and the emergence of lifespan psychology (Baltes, Staudinger, & Lindenberger, 1999) that kept wisdom in the domain of psychological analysis. Starting in the 1980s, a more diverse group of scholars and researchers began to engage themselves with the topic of wisdom, although most work was theoretical rather than empirical (Baltes & Staudinger, 2000).

Due to the multidisciplinary nature of the wisdom concept, psychological research on wisdom is multifaceted (Baltes & Staudinger, 2000), and there is as yet no generally agreed upon definition of wisdom (Ardelt, 2004). Sternberg (1998) differentiated three major approaches to understanding wisdom. The approaches are classified as philosophical, implicit theoretical, and explicit theoretical approaches.

Philosophical perspectives on wisdom

The study of wisdom has a history that long antedates psychological study, with the Platonic dialogues offering the first intensive Western analysis of the concept of wisdom (Sternberg, 1998). Plato pointed out that the assignment of human intelligence is to become wise. Thus the virtue of intelligence is wisdom (Kunzmann, Burkard, Wiedman, 1998). Robinson (1990) identified three different meanings of wisdom in the platonic dialogues: wisdom as (a) sophia, which is found in those who seek a contemplative life in search of truth; (b) phronesis, which is the kind of practical wisdom shown by statesmen and legislators; and (c) episteme, which is found in those who understand things from a scientific point of view. Aristotle distinguished between phronesis, the kind of practical wisdom mentioned above, and theoretikes, which is theoretical knowledge devoted to truth (Sternberg, 1998). Robinson (1989) argued that, according to Aristotle, a wise individual knows more than the material, efficient, or formal causes behind an event.

Many other philosophical conceptions of wisdom (for an overview see Robinson, 1990) have followed the early Greek ones. An example can be seen in most modern religions, which aim for wisdom conceptualized as an understanding not just of the material world, but also of the spiritual world and its relationships to the material world (Sternberg, 1998).

Implicit theoretical approaches

Implicit approaches to wisdom refer to folk psychological or common sense approaches and the use of "wisdom" in everyday language (Baltes & Staudinger, 2000). This line of work was initiated by Clayton (1975, 1976, 1982; Clayton & Birren, 1980), who identified two consistent dimensions in the implicit conceptions of wisdom in adult laypersons: an affective dimension, and a reflective dimension.

Holliday and Chandler (1986) identified five factors underlying the folk concept of wisdom: exceptional understanding, judgment and communication skills, general competence, interpersonal skills, and social unobtrusiveness.

In a series of studies investigating implicit theories of wisdom, Sternberg (1985) identified six components that accounted for wisdom: reasoning ability, sagacity, learning from ideas and environment, judgment, expeditious use of information, and perspicacity.

Baltes and Staudinger (2000) drew five conclusions from the results of implicit conceptions of wisdom and wise persons: a) Wisdom is a concept that carries specific meaning that is widely shared and understood in its language-based representation. b) Wisdom is judged to be an exceptional level of human functioning. c) Wisdom identifies a state of mind and behavior that includes the coordinated and balanced interplay of intellectual, affective, and motivational aspects of human functioning. d) Wisdom is viewed as associated with a high degree of personal and interpersonal competence. e) Wisdom involves good intentions.

Consistent with the view that implicit and folk psychological characterizations of wisdom are mainly the product of cultural history and its impact on current society is the view that a more comprehensive characterization of wisdom can be deduced from cultural-historical and philosophical analyses of the wisdom concept. Baltes (1993) utilized such a cultural-historical and philosophical analysis in order to obtain a more general and comprehensive conceptualization of wisdom (see also Baltes and Staudinger, 2000). Table 3 illustrates seven properties of wisdom.

Table 3. General criteria outlining the nature of wisdom derived from cultural-historical analysis (cf. Baltes & Staudinger, 2000, p. 135)

- Wisdom addresses important and difficult questions and strategies
  about the conduct and meaning of life.

- Wisdom includes knowledge about the limits of knowledge and the
  uncertainties of the world.

- Wisdom represents a truly superior level of knowledge, judgment, and
  advice.

- Wisdom constitutes knowledge with extraordinary scope, depth, measure, and balance.

- Wisdom involves a perfect synergy of mind and character, that is, an
  orchestration of knowledge and virtues.

- Wisdom represents knowledge used for the good or well-being of oneself and others.

- Wisdom is easily recognized when manifested, although difficult to
  achieve and to specify.

Explicit theoretical approaches

Whereas implicit theories are based on the beliefs and mental representations of
everyday persons about wisdom and wise people, explicit theories are constructs
of (supposedly) expert theorists and researchers (Ardelt, 2004). Most explicit
theories are based on constructs from the psychology of human development
(Sternberg, 1998).

In extending the Piagetian stages of intelligence (Piaget, 1972), some theorists viewed wisdom in terms of postformal operational thinking. Kitchener
and Brenner (1990) stated that wisdom requires a synthesis of knowledge from
opposing points of view. In accordance, Labouvie-Vief (1990) emphasized
the importance of a smooth and balanced dialogue between logical forms of
processing and more subjective forms of processing. Pascual-Leone (1990)
emphasized the importance of the integration of all aspects of a person's affect,
cognition, motivation, and life experience. The importance of the integration of
relativistic and dialectic modes of thinking, affect, and reflection was emphasized by Kramer (1990). In reference to a number of views on wisdom, Birren
and Fisher (1990) also suggested the importance of the integration of cognitive,
conative, and affective aspects of human abilities.

Other theorists have stressed the importance of knowing the limits of one's own extant knowledge and of then trying to go beyond them (Sternberg, 1998). Meacham (1990), for example, emphasized that an important aspect of wisdom is an awareness of one's own fallibility and knowledge of what one does and does not know. Similarly, Kitchener and Brenner (1990) stressed the importance of knowing the limitations of one's own knowledge.

An elaborated psychological theory of wisdom was put forward by Sternberg (1998). Sternberg conceptualized wisdom as the application of tacit knowledge toward the achievement of a common good through a balance among multiple personal (intra-, inter-, and extrapersonal) interests and environmental conditions. In this view, wisdom is a subset of practical intelligence applied in particular to seek good ends for oneself (intrapersonal interests), at the same time balancing them with good outcomes for others (interpersonal interests) and with the contextual factors (extrapersonal interests) involved.

A relatively parsimonious model of wisdom was suggested by Ardelt (2004). In her view, wisdom is an integration of cognitive, reflective, and affective personality characteristics. The cognitive dimension of wisdom refers to an understanding of life and a desire to know the truth, particularly with regard to intrapersonal and interpersonal matters. This includes knowledge and acceptance of the positive and negative aspects of human nature, of the inherent limits of knowledge, and of life's unpredictability and uncertainties. The reflective component of wisdom represents self-examination, self-awareness, self-insight, and the ability to look at phenomena and events from different perspectives. The affective component consists of a person's sympathetic and compassionate love for others (Ardelt, 2004, 2005). In order to assess the three personality characteristics of wisdom, Ardelt (2003) developed a standardized self-report questionnaire, the three-dimensional wisdom scale (3D-WS).

Most developmental approaches to wisdom are ontogenetic. However, Csikszentmihalyi and Rathunde (1990) have taken a philogenetic or evolutionary approach, arguing that constructs such as wisdom must have been selected over time, at least in a cultural sense. From this point of view, wise ideas should survive better over time than unwise ideas in a culture (Sternberg, 1998).

The Berlin wisdom paradigm

Baltes and colleagues (Baltes & Smith, 1990; Baltes & Staudinger, 1993; Baltes & Staudinger, 2000) have developed the most prominent and extensive empirical program dedicated to the study of wisdom (Ardelt, 2004; Sternberg, 1998). Even though this program does not cover the entire meaning space of wisdom, it does allow the operationalization and measurement of wisdom-related behavior (Baltes & Staudinger, 2000).

Based on cultural-historical and philosophical analyses of the wisdom concept (see Table 3) Baltes and colleagues define wisdom as "an expertise in the conduct and meaning of life" (Baltes and Staudinger, 2000, p.124), and as "expert knowledge in the fundamental pragmatics of life that permits exceptional insight, judgment, and advice about complex and uncertain matters" (Baltes & Smith, 1990, p. 95). As can be seen from these definitions, an emphasis of wisdom is put on excellence, and the term wisdom is reserved to only denote the highest levels of performance. Thus it is assumed that eliciting wisdom puts extremely high demands on knowledge and judgment. In this vein, lower performance levels are labeled wisdom related (Staudinger & Baltes, 1996b).

The concept of fundamental pragmatics of life refers to knowledge and judgment about the quintessential aspects of the human condition, including its biological boundaries, cultural conditioning, and variability both within and across individuals (Baltes & Staudinger, 2000; Pasupathi, Staudinger, & Baltes, 2001). Wisdom concerns the essential aspects of life, and is used for the good of oneself and others and is applied in the planning, management, and interpretation of human lives (Pasupathi, et al. 2001).

In contrast to other wisdom researchers, the Berlin group does not conceptualize wisdom as a personality characteristic or a combination of personality qualities, but as an expert knowledge system. Wisdom as a body of knowledge concerning the conduct, interpretation, and meaning of life is seen as a cultural and collective product (Baltes & Staudinger, 2000). Thus the focus of the Berlin group's work is on wisdom-related knowledge rather than wise individuals. In reference to Western philosophical analyses of wisdom, the aim was to define wisdom on a theoretical and abstract level, and to subsequently study how people can be described within the theory's framework (Baltes & Kunzmann, 2004). In this regard, individuals are considered to be imperfect carriers of the collectively anchored product wisdom (Baltes & Staudinger, 2000; Baltes & Kunzmann, 2004). The theoretical framework suggested by the Berlin group allows to sort individuals into levels of wisdom and to examine the conditions that produce interindividual differences (Baltes & Kunzmann, 2004).

Five criteria, i.e., factual knowledge, procedural knowledge, lifespan contextualism, value relativism, recognition and management of uncertainty (see Table 4) have been outlined to assess the quality and quantity of wisdom-related performance in individuals (Baltes & Smith, 1990; Staudinger & Baltes, 1996a, 1996b). The two general, basic wisdom criteria factual and procedural knowledge are derived from general conceptions of expert systems (e.g., Chi, Glaser, & Rees, 1982; Ericsson & Smith, 1991). Applied to the field of wisdom research, these criteria are: (1) Rich factual (declarative) knowledge about the fundamental pragmatics of life. This part "concerns knowledge about such topics as human nature, life-long development, variations in developmental processes and outcomes, interpersonal relations, social norms, critical events in life and their possible constellations, as well as knowledge about the coordination of the well-being of oneself and that of others." (2) Rich procedural knowledge about the fundamental pragmatics of life. This part "involves strategies and heuristics for giving advice and for the structuring and weighing of life goals, ways to handle life conflicts and life decisions, and knowledge about alternative back-up strategies if development were not to proceed as expected" (Baltes and Staudinger, 2000, p. 125). The two basic wisdom criteria are considered to be necessary but not sufficient to define wisdom-related performance (Pasupathi, et al. 2001).

The three remaining criteria are metalevel or meta-criteria and are considered to be, in their separate and joint expression, specific to wisdom (Baltes & Staudinger, 2000). They are grounded in analyses of the ancient wisdom literature, neo-Piagetian research on postformal thought, and propositions put forward by lifespan developmental psychology (Staudinger & Baltes, 1996b). The first meta-criterion, (3) lifespan contextualism, "is meant to identify knowledge that considers the many themes and contexts in life (e.g., education, family, work, friends, leisure, the public good of society, etc.), their interrelations and cultural variations, and in addition, incorporates a lifetime temporal perspective (i.e., past, present, and future) " (Baltes & Staudinger, 2000, p. 125/126). (4) Value relativism, the second meta-criterion, deals with the acknowledgment of and tolerance for value differences and the relativity of the values held by individuals and society, while simultaneously recognizing certain universal values that promote the common and individual good. The third meta-criterion, (5) recognition and management of uncertainty, refers to an awareness and management of the inherent uncertainty of individual and collective life (Baltes & Staudinger, 2000).

The focus of the Berlin group, to date, has primarily been on manifestations of wisdom in individual minds. In order to elicit and measure wisdom-related knowledge and skills, individuals are confronted with various difficult life dilemmas of fictitious people, such as the following examples, under standardized conditions (method of irresolvable problems; Baltes & Staudinger, 2000, p. 126):

Someone receives a telephone call from a good friend who says that he or she cannot go on like this and has decided to commit suicide. What might one/the person take into consideration and do in such a situation?

In reflecting over their lives, people sometimes realize that they have not achieved what they had once planned to achieve. What should they do and consider?

Table 4. Five criteria characterizing wisdom and wisdom-related performance (cf. Staudinger & Baltes, 1996b, p. 747)

Criteria	Key evaluation question
Basic	
Factual knowledge	To what extent does this performance show general (*condition humana*) and specific (e.g., life events, variations, institutions) knowledge about life matters as well as demonstrate scope and depth in the coverage of issues?
Procedural knowledge	To what extend does this performance consider strategies of decision making (e.g., cost-benefit analysis), self-regulation, life-interpretation, life-planning (e.g., means-ends analysis), and advice giving (e.g., timing, withholding)?
Meta-level	
Lifespan contextualism	To what extend does this performance consider the past, current, and possible future contexts of life and the many circumstances (e.g., culturally graded, age graded, idiosyncratic) in which a life is embedded and how they relate to each other?
Value relativism	To what extend does this performance consider variations in values and life priorities and the importance to view each person within his or her own framework of values and life-goals, despite a small set of universal values such as the orientation toward the well-being of oneself and others?
Recognition and management of uncertainty	To what extend does this performance consider the inherent uncertainty of life (in terms of interpreting the past, predicting the future, managing the present) and effective strategies for dealing with uncertainty (e.g., back-up solutions, optimizing gain-loss ratio)?

Participants are then asked to reflect out loud on the presented dilemma, and the responses are recorded on tape and transcribed. Before the tasks are administered, participants are trained in thinking aloud and thinking about a hypothetical person. In order to obtain quantified scores, a selected panel of trained judges evaluates the protocols of the respondents in light of the five wisdom-related criteria (see Table 4) using a 7-point scale. The reliability of this rating method has been proven to be very satisfactory (Baltes & Staudinger, 2000). Table 5 shows a high- and low-rated response to the question of what to consider and do in the case of a 15-year-old girl who wants to get married right away.

Table 5. Wisdom-related task with examples of extreme responses (abbreviated) (cf. Baltes & Staudinger, 2000, p. 136)

A 15-year-old girl wants to get married right away. What should one/she consider and do?	
Low wisdom-related score	A 15-year-old girl who wants to get married? No, no way. Marrying at age 15 would be utterly wrong. One has to tell the girl that marriage is not possible. (After further probing) It would be irresponsible to support such an idea. No, this is just a crazy idea.
High wisdom-related score	Well, on the surface, this seems like an easy problem. On average, marriage for 15-year-old girls is not a good thing. But there are situations where the average case does not fit. Perhaps in this instance, special life circumstances are involved, such that the girl has a terminal illness. Or the girl has just lost her parents. And also, this girl may live in another culture or historical period. Perhaps she was raised with a value system different from ours. In addition, one has to think about adequate ways of talking with the girl and to consider her emotional state.

A wide range of data collected by Baltes and colleagues demonstrate the empirical usefulness of the proposed theoretical and measurement approaches to wisdom (e.g., Baltes, Smith and Staudinger, 1992; Baltes & Staudinger, 1993). Staudinger, Lopez, and Baltes (1997) found that measures of intelligence and personality as well as their interface overlap with but are not identical to measures of wisdom in terms of constructs measured. Thus, wisdom-related performance evinced a fair degree of measurement independence (uniqueness). Furthermore, no major age differences in wisdom-related performance were found for the age range from about 25 to 75 years of age (Smith & Baltes, 1990; Staudinger & Baltes, 1996a; Staudinger, 1999). These findings support the idea that wisdom-related knowledge and judgment are facets of human development that do not show signs of deterioration with increasing age. Moreover, it shows that having lived longer in itself is not sufficient for acquiring more knowledge and judgment capacity in the wisdom-related domain (Baltes & Staudinger, 2000).

In addition, Ardelt (1997) demonstrated that wisdom (defined as a composite of cognitive, reflective, and affective qualities)[8] has a profoundly positive influence on life satisfaction in women and men independent of objective circumstances. Moreover, it was shown that wisdom can help to compensate the impact of negative events. These findings are supported by Lyster (1996) and Bacelar (1998) who showed that wisdom is a better predictor of life satisfaction than objective circumstances. On these grounds, it is no surprise that wisdom and wisdom-related knowledge are currently regarded as an objective of therapeutic interventions (Maercker, 1997). Especially since there is evidence that wisdom-related knowledge can be activated by cognitive interventions (Böhmig-Krumhaar, 1998).

Wisdom and coping with negative life events

Wise people are considered to be capable of dealing with any crisis and obstacle that they encounter (Ardelt, 2000a; 2000b; 2005; Assman, 1994; Baltes & Freund, 2003; Baltes & Kunzmann, 2003; Bianachi, 1994; Clayton, 1982; Dittmann-Kohli & Baltes, 1990; Kekes, 1983, 1995; Kramer, 2000; Kunzmann & Baltes, 2003; Sternberg, 1998; Vaillant, 1993). However, only one study (Ardelt, 2005) to date has analyzed what wise individuals actually do when confronted with hardship and obstacles in life.

In an exploratory qualitive study, Ardelt (2005) examined coping strategies of three individuals with relatively high wisdom scores on the three-dimensional wisdom scale (3D-WS) (see Ardelt, 2003). Three higher-order strategies were identified and summarized as mental distancing, active coping, and application of life lessons.

When confronted with a crisis, relatively wise individuals took a step back, calmed down, and reflected on the situation from an emotional distance (mental distancing). Furthermore, they often mentally redefined problems as challenging or interesting rather than unpleasant, in order to take control of the situation (active coping). In addition, they were not devastated by crisis and hardship in their life. On the contrary, they were able to learn from negative experiences. They learned to accept that life is unpredictable and uncertain, with the result that they were better prepared to face new crises and obstacles (application of

---

[8] Ardelt (1997) used a different conceptualization of wisdom than the Berlin group (see the section on assessment of cognitive and emotional wisdom below).

life lessons). In contrast, persons relatively low on wisdom did allow external events to take possession of their being. They did not recognize that it is ultimately not the external event that affects their well-being, but how they react to and deal with crises and hardships in their lives. These findings indicate that wisdom comprises competencies that allow an individual to efficiently cope with negative life events and crises. Thus, a lack in wisdom-related knowledge can be seen as a vulnerability factor for reactive disorders, which develop in response to a variety of stressful events, the symptoms representing a maladaptation to these stressors (Casey et al. 2001).

Change of perspective

Ardelt (2003) argues that an additional component of wisdom is the ability to change perspectives, that is, to understand the world from the position of others. It describes the degree to which a person is capable and willing to look at events from different perspectives. Recognition and understanding of views, interests, motives, and situational constraints of other people can facilitate an understanding of their behavior and of emerging conflicts. In behavior therapy, change of perspective is trained by means of role change techniques.

Wisdom in a clinical context

As discussed above, the Berlin group does not conceptualize wisdom as a personality characteristic or a combination of personality qualities, but as a cultural and collective product and as an expertise (Baltes & Staudinger, 2000). Thus, the focus is on wisdom-related knowledge rather than wise individuals. The Berlin group specifically does not ask respondents to evaluate their own life or how they have solved their own problems or those of family and friends. The reason is their interest "in subjects' general knowledge of the domain, fundamental pragmatics of life, rather than in the way they have applied this knowledge to themselves" (Smith & Baltes, 1990, p. 495).

This concept allows to ask for wisdom also in a clinical context. Important questions are a) What is the degree of "wisdom expertise" in a person? Low levels could be seen as a vulnerability factor which can hinder coping with negative life events and lead to dysfunctional reactions. b) Is the degree of wisdom in a person sufficient to cope with a given exceptional life event? Different life events require different degrees of coping capacities. Extreme life events may still be mastered when very high rates of wisdom are given, or normal rates of wisdom may no longer be sufficient. c) Can wisdom expertise be trained and enhanced, when more wisdom is needed? This could be the starting point for a new psychotherapeutic avenue.

Emotional Intelligence

Cognition and Emotion

The meaning of life events is mediated by cognitions, i.e., meanings of the event, interpretations, or attributions of values. These are directly associated with emotional reactions. Whenever patients with PTED think about the trigger event, concomitant emotions like embitterment are felt and can become very strong. In the end, emotions are the pivotal problem, as they in turn stimulate emotion-dependent cognitions.

Therefore, dealing with a critical event requires not only cognitive abilities, but emotional ones as well. The application of wisdom-related knowledge when confronted with a negative life event that involves personal consternation requires the ability to perceive, understand, and manage (negative) emotions regarding oneself and others. Thus, in accordance with the "intrapersonal interests" of Sternberg (1989) and Ardelt (2003), cognitive dimensions of wisdom must be accompanied by "emotional wisdom." This aspect of emotional involvement and consternation in reaction to a negative life event is recognized in reference to the theory of "emotional intelligence" by Mayer & Salovey (e.g. Mayer & Salovey, 1995, 1997; Mayer, Salovey, Caruso, 2004) and the three-dimensional model of wisdom by Ardelt (2003; 2004; see also above).

Emotional intelligence

Emotional intelligence is a psychological concept that has received much attention not only in science but also in the general public with often unclear definitions and little empirical substance (Matthews, Zeidner, & Roberts, 2002, Matthews, Roberts &, Zeidner, 2004). The best-defined and elaborated operationalization of emotional intelligence has been put forward by Mayer & Salovey (e.g., 1995, 1997; Salovey & Mayer, 1990). They define EI as:

the capacity to reason about emotions, and of emotions to enhance thinking. It includes the abilities to accurately perceive emotions, to access and generate emotions so as to assist thought, to understand emotions and emotional knowledge, and to reflectively regulate emotions so as to promote emotional and intellectual growth (Mayer, Salovey, & Caruso, 2004, p. 197).

From this perspective, emotional intelligence is understood as a member of a class of intelligences including the social, practical, and personal intelligences that are called the hot intelligences. The label hot refers to the fact that these intelligences operate on cognitions dealing with matters of personal, emotional importance to the individual (Abelson, 1963; Zajonc, 1980). Thus, emotional intelligence is conceived as operating on emotional information. Individuals with high emotional intelligence are considered to better perceive emotions, use them in thought, understand their meanings, and manage emotions better than others. Solving emotional problems likely requires less cognitive effort for these individuals (Mayer, Salovey, & Caruso, 2004). Overall, emotional competencies as summarized by this concept are a prerequisite to successful coping with negative events that are personal and highly emotional.

With reference to the concept of emotional intelligence by Mayer & Salovey (1995, 1997), and in regard of our clinical experience with PTED patients, we chose four dimensions to describe and assess "emotional components of wisdom":
  - perception and acceptance of emotions,
  - empathy,
  - serenity, and
  - long-term perspective.

"Perception and acceptance of emotions" are necessary to solve or cope with problems dealing with matters of personal and emotional importance to the individual. Coping with emotionally loaded problems requires the ability to accurately identify emotions and the ability to distinguish between different emotions (Baumann et al., 2005). Perception of emotions, particularly the perception of negative emotions, also depends on the willingness to accept them. Patients with PTED tend to disclaim negative and undesirable emotions. Especially, "unacceptable" emotions like anger, humiliation, and thoughts of revenge are often denied because they contradict moral beliefs. Hence, the willingness to accept emotions is incorporated into our conceptualization of wisdom.

"Empathy" is needed to solve or cope with interpersonal problems (e.g., marital problems, conflicts with the boss, or the like). In our concept empathy is understood as an "emotional change of perspective." It is the ability to recognize and emphasize emotions of the other persons.

"Serenity" is the ability to control one's emotions and to have and show functional instead of dysfunctional emotions. When coping with different problems, different emotions can be helpful or harmful. Solutions can be facilitated by some emotions but not others (Izard, 2001, Erez & Isen, 2002; Isen, 2001; Palfai & Salovey, 1993). Serenity, therefore, refers to the ability to manage emotions so that they help to solve problems or reach certain goals. That is, emotions are managed in the context of the individual's goals, self-knowledge, and social awareness (Mayer, Salovey, & Caruso, 2004).

"Long-term perspective" refers to the ability to delay gratification. This is a capacity which has been found to be related to the subsequent development of intellectual and emotional competences already in 4-year-old children (Shoda, Mischel and Peake, 1990). Furthermore, it has been shown that the ability to delay gratification, independently of intelligence, reinforced intellectual performance (Goleman, 1999). From this perspective, the ability to delay gratification can be understood as a meta-ability, which determines to what extent an individual is able to use their mental capacities. A similar concept can be found in behavior therapy which makes a distinction between short- and long-term successful behavior. Behavior which is associated with short-term success (shouting at somebody) is often dysfunctional in the long run (withdrawal of friends). From this perspective, the pursuit of long-term strategies requires the management of negative emotions, which rather motivate the pursuit of short-term strategies.

Assessment of cognitive and emotional wisdom

The summary of theories on wisdom and emotional intelligence shows that wisdom is a set of different kinds of expertise and not a one-dimensional construct. This makes operationalization and measurement difficult. In the Berlin Wisdom Project, wisdom was measured by using the paradigm of reasoning on complex life problems. Participants were asked to imagine that their very young daughter wanted to marry and to discuss how to react. Their answers were then rated as more or less wise on the five dimensions: factual (declarative) knowledge about the fundamental pragmatics of life, procedural knowledge about the fundamental pragmatics of life, lifespan contextualism, value relativism, and recognition and management of uncertainty (Baltes & Staudinger, 2000).

Following this model and referring to the theoretical concepts of wisdom and emotional intelligence, we developed a set of nine dimensions to assess cognitive and emotional wisdom expertise (see also Table 6):

1. change of perspective,
2. empathy,
3. perception and acceptance of emotions,
4. serenity,
5. factual knowledge,
6. contextualism,
7. value relativism,
8. uncertainty acceptance, and
9. long-term perspective.

Table 6. Dimensions of cognitive and emotional wisdom-related expertise

Criteria	Key evaluation question
Change of perspective	To what extent does this performance show that the different perspectives of the persons concerned are recognized?
Empathy	To what extend does this performance show that the emotions of the different persons concerned are recognized and empathized with?
Perception and acceptance of emotions	To what extend does this performance show that one's own emotions are recognized and accepted?
Serenity	To what extend does this performance show that different perspectives and arguments are reported in an emotionally balanced way?
Factual knowledge and procedural knowledge	To what extent does this performance show general and specific (e.g., life events, variations, institutions) knowledge about life matters and consider strategies of decision making (e.g., cost-benefit analysis) and problem solving?
Contextualism	To what extend does this performance consider the past, current, and possible future contexts of life and the many circumstances in which a life is embedded?
Value relativism	To what extend does this performance consider variations in values and life priorities and the importance of viewing each person within his or her own framework of values and life-goals, despite a small set of universal values?
Uncertainty acceptance	To what extend does this performance consider the inherent uncertainty of life (in terms of interpreting the past, predicting the future, managing the present) and effective strategies for dealing with uncertainty?
Long-term perspective	To what extent does this performance consider that each behavior can have positive and negative, as well as short- and long-term consequences, which can also contradict each other?

Participants are given life problems which have no simple solution and can be characterized as unjust: "Mr. Smith is imprisoned because he is accused of fraud. After six months, his innocence is proven and he is discharged. Meanwhile his wife has left him." The participants are then asked to reflect out loud on the problem presented. Specifically, they are asked what they would consider and do if they were Mr. Smith. Wisdom-related expertise can be rated on each of the nine dimensions using a global judgment on a five-point scale ranging from "not at all" (0) to "very much" (4). Apart from such general and fictitious problems, patients can also be asked to comment on their personal life problem.

This cognitive-emotional-wisdom-expertise rating (CEWE-rating) allows for the study of degrees of wisdom expertise in the context of adjustment disorders and can also serve as a guide for the training of wisdom expertise.

2. Empirical Evidence

The concept of PTED has been developed on the basis of clinical observations and problems with the treatment of such patients. After the first description of the clinical concept of PTED (Linden, 2003), a pilot study was conducted (Linden et al. 2004), including 21 patients who were clinically judged to suffer from PTED and who suffered from a variety of psychopathological signs and symptoms and were severely impaired in their daily lives. This study helped to define diagnostic criteria and set up a diagnostic interview. These were then tested in a larger study in which PTED patients were compared with a matched sample of patients with other mental disorders. Additionally, a number of further studies were done to develop a self-rating scale and get initial epidemiological data. This second part of this book summarizes the empirical findings of these studies on PTED and also gives details on instruments for the assessment of PTED.

2.1 The Psychopathology of PTED

PTED patients and controls

In order to study the psychopathological features of patients with PTED, all patients in the Department of Behavioral Medicine and Psychosomatics of the Rehabilitation Center Seehof were screened. Out of approximately 1,200 inpatients, 96 were reported as possibly suffering from PTED by the treating physicians. 88 of these were interviewed by a study physician, who made a diagnosis of PTED according to clinical judgment in 50 patients (30 women, 20 men). In addition, a control group of 50 patients was recruited who were treated as inpatients because of other mental disorders (control group). Whenever a PTED patient was admitted, the next incoming patient with the same gender and age was selected for the control group. All patients of the control group were classified as non-PTED patients according to the clinical assessment by the study physician.

Table 7 gives an overview of socio-demographic characteristics of both samples. Gender distribution and age were the same in both samples (60%

Table 7. Sociodemographic data of PTED and control patients

	PTED sample % resp. mean (SD) $n = 50$	Control group % resp. mean (SD) $n = 50$	*t*-test resp. χ^2	Significance
Female	60.0%	60.0%	$\chi^2 = 0.000$	$p = 1.000$
Age (years)	49.7 (6.98)	49.4 (6.69)	$t(98) = -.190$	$p = 0.850$
Married	77,6%	64.0%	$\chi^2 = 2.194$	$p = 0.139$
Permanent job	46.9%	87.5%	$\chi^2 = 11.978$	$p = 0.001$
Premorbid Intelligence (MWT-B[9])	110 (14.78)	112 (14.6)	$t(68) = .653$	$p = 0.517$

Note. Missing Data: For *Married*: PTED patients $n = 49$. For *Permanent job*: $n = 32$ for both groups. For *IQ*: PTED patients $n = 39$; Control group $n = 31$.

---

9 Note that the MWT-B overestimates general intelligence. In healthy subjects, the MWT-B resulted on average in an IQ 17 points higher than the Verbal and 16 points higher than the Full Scale IQ of the HAWIE-R, the German equivalent of the Wechsler Adult Intelligence Scale-R (Satzger, Fessmann, Engel, 2002).

women; mean age: 49), due to the matching of participants. No differences ($\chi^2 = 2.194$, $p = .13$) were found between the groups with regard to family status or intelligence. A significant difference between the groups was found in occupational status ($\chi^2 = 11.978$, $p = .001$). 87.5% of the control group had a permanent job, compared to 46.9% of the PTED sample.

After recruitment, each participant was examined with the Mini International Neuropsychiatric Interview in the German version 4.4 (MINI; Sheehan, Lecrubier, Janavs et al. 1994) and a standardized interview on PTED criteria and psychopathological features. Patients also filled in the Bern Embitterment Questionnaire (Znoj, 2002), the Symptom-Checklist-90-Revision (SCL-90-R; Franke, 1995), and the Impact of Event Scale (IES-R) in the modification published by Maercker & Schützwohl (1998).

Psychiatric diagnoses in PTED patients and controls

Table 8 shows the spectrum of psychiatric diagnoses on the basis of the MINI psychiatric interview (MINI; Sheehan, Lecrubier, Janavs et al. 1994). Chi-square tests were calculated to test for significant differences. Both groups fulfilled the criteria for many disorders with a significantly higher occurrence of major depression ($\chi^2 = 16.88$, $p < .001$) and chronic adjustment disorder ($\chi^2 = 21.58$, $p < .001$), but less generalized anxiety disorder lifetime ($\chi^2 = 7.16$, $p = .007$) in PTED patients. In total, criteria for 192 diagnoses were fulfilled in the control group, and 212 in the PTED group.

These findings indicate a high degree of comorbidity and/or diagnostic uncertainty in PTED. The most frequent diagnoses were adjustment disorder (66%), major depression (50%), dysthymia (40%), generalized anxiety disorder (34%), social phobia (18%), agoraphobia (18%), and personality disorder (16%). Although patients complained about multiple somatic symptoms, no diagnosis of a somatization disorder could be made, because the diagnostic criteria were not met (age over 30, many somatic complaints over several years, onset of complaints before the age of 30, strong influence on everyday life).

Phenomenology of PTED

All PTED patients reported at least one critical event which they experienced as unjust and insulting. Forty-eight saw this event as the direct cause of their present state and of a persistent negative change in their well-being. As a core criterion in the concept of PTED is that the patient has experienced his present

Table 8. Diagnostic spectrum according to the MINI standardized interview
($N = 100$)

	Embittered patients % ($n = 50$)	Control group % ($n = 50$)	p χ^2
Major depression (acute)	50.0	12.0	0.001***
Major depression (lifetime)	44.0	60.0	0.109
Dysthymia (acute)	40.0	24.0	0.086
Dysthymia (lifetime)	4.0	10.0	0.436
Hypomanic periods (acute)	0.0	0.0	
Hypomanic periods (lifetime)	6.0	14.0	0.182
Manic periods (acute)	0	0	
Manic periods (lifetime)	0	0	
Panic disorder (acute)	12.0	6.0	0.487
Panic disorder (lifetime)	0	0	
Panic disorder with few symptoms (acute)	10.0	6.0	0.715
Panic disorder with few symptoms (lifetime)	2.0	4.0	1.000
Agoraphobia (acute)	18.0	14.0	0.585
Agoraphobia (lifetime)	4.0	4.0	1.000
Social phobia (acute)	18.0	14.0	0.585
Social phobia (lifetime)	0.0	6.0	0.242
OCD (acute)	4.0	4.0	1.000
OCD (lifetime)	0.0	2.0	0.495
Generalized anxiety disorder (acute)	34.0	28.0	0.517
Generalized anxiety disorder (lifetime)	4.0	22.0	0.007**
Alcohol addiction (acute)	6.0	10.0	0.715
Alcohol abuse (acute)	2.0	2.0	1.000
Alcohol addiction (lifetime)	2.0	8.0	0.362
Alcohol abuse (lifetime)	2.0	0.0	1.000
Drug addiction (acute)	2.0	2.0	1.000

Table 8. (continued)

	Embittered patients % ($n = 50$)	Control group % ($n = 50$)	p χ^2
Drug abuse (acute)	0.0	2.0	1.000
Drug addiction (lifetime)	0.0	6.0	0.242
Drug abuse (lifetime)	0.0	0.0	
Psychosis (acute)	0.0	0.0	
Psychosis (lifetime)	0.0	0.0	
Affective disorder with psychotic signs	0.0	0.0	
Anorexia nervosa (acute)	0.0	0.0	
Affective disorder with psychotic signs	0.0	0.0	
Anorexia nervosa (acute)	0.0	0.0	
Anorexia nervosa (lifetime)	0.0	0.0	
Bulimia (acute)	2.0	0.0	1.000
Anorexia nervosa/type bulimia (acute)	0.0	0.0	
Bulimia (lifetime)	2.0	0.0	1.000
Suicidal (acute)	20.0	14.3	0.451
Suicidal (lifetime)	36.0	34.7	0.892
PTSD (acute)	2.0	2.0	1.000
PTSD (lifetime)	4.0	12.0	0.269
Somatization (lifetime)	2.0	2.0	1.000
Somatization (acute)	0.0	0.0	
Adjustment disorder (acute)	0.0	2.0	1.000
Adjustment disorder (lifetime)	66.0	20.0	0.001***
Personality disorder	16.0	22.0	0.444
Mixed anxiety/depression (acute)	2.0	0.0	1.000
Hypochondriasis (acute)	2.0	2.0	1.000
Hypochondriasis (lifetime)	2.0	10.0	0.204

negative state as a direct consequence of the negative life event, the two patients who did not make this statement were excluded from the following analysis.[10] No preexisting mental disorders or personality disorders were detected, looking at the history of the patients.

The reported critical life events were work related in 72.9% of patients, related to the family or partnership in 12.5%, in 8.3% it was the death of a relative or a friend, and in 6.3% an illness. Most frequently reported events related to work were job loss or mobbing. These findings suggest that negative live events in the work-related context play a prominent role in PTED. But one has to take into account that the sample consisted of patients of a rehabilitation clinic where the majority of patients are treated for work-related incapacities. Different distributions of critical events may be seen in other populations.

Duration of illness

The duration of illness (see Figure 1) ranged from 6 to 144 months (Mean = 31.7; SD = 35.5) at the time of examination. Thus, the duration of PTED exceeds the defined duration of 6 months for adjustment disorder. In about one third of the cases (31.3%) the duration of illness was longer then 2 years, in 6 cases (12.5%), the duration was 5 years and longer.

Figure 1. Duration of PTED (*n* = 48)

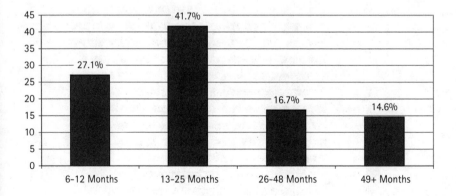

---

10 The possible reasons for the fact that two of the clinically defined PTED patients did not meet the criteria for PTED will be discussed in more detail in chapter 2.2.

Psychopathological and emotional spectrum in PTED

Looking at psychopathological signs and symptoms in more detail (see Figure 2), all patients reported that they had been suffering from intrusive thoughts and memories of the event during the previous months; 97.9% of the patients complained of persistent negative mood, and 91.7% of restlessness since the critical event; 77.1% of the patients avoided places and people which remind them of the event; 75% confirmed a general feeling of resignation since the event and stated that there would be no meaning in further effort; 83.3% complained about a loss of interest, 83.3% about inhibition, and 79.2% about early awakening, symptoms which are typically seen in melancholic depression. But different from melancholic depression, 91.7% said that they were able to experience normal affect when distracted.

When asked for emotions which patients experience when reminded of the critical event (see Figure 3), all patients reported that they had experienced the critical event as unjust and unfair. Furthermore, they said to feel embitterment (97.7%), rage (91.7%), helplessness (91.7%), and anger (85.4%). 85.1% said they would welcome it if the person responsible were called to account. In addition, a general decline in social activities was found. 79.2% of the patients

Figure 2. Psychopathological spectrum in connection with the critical event ($n = 48$)

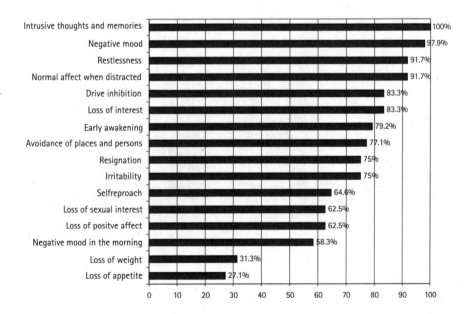

Figure 3. Emotional spectrum in connection with the critical event (*n* = 48)

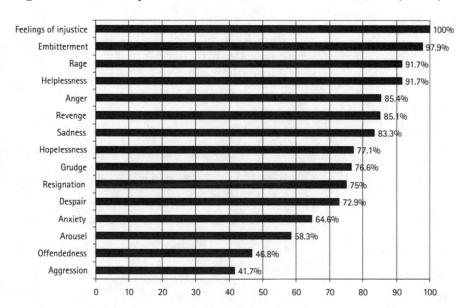

indicated a reduction in their occupational activities, 75% a reduction in leisure time activities, and 54.2% a reduction in family activities.

Self-assessment of PTED and control patients

To compare both patient groups, all participants were asked to fill in a set of self-report questionnaires. The results of the SCL-90-R, the IES-R, and the Bern Embitterment questionnaire are summarized in Table 9. Due to the subsequent inclusion of the IES-R, and because of missing data, the sample sizes differ between instruments.

Clear differences were found between the two patient groups with regard to the quality and intensity of psychopathological symptoms. The SCL-90-R indicated that PTED patients report markedly more severe symptoms than the control group. The PTED group scored significantly higher on the Global Severity Index (Total score = 1.13 vs. 0.74; $\Delta = 0.39$; t (97) = -3.71, $P < .001$), the Positive Symptom Total (TS = 52.22 vs. 39.30; $\Delta = 12.92$; t (97) = -3.49, $P = .001$), and the Positive Symptom Distress Index (TS = 1.86 vs. 1.57; $\Delta = 0.29$; t (97) = -3.18, $P = .002$), as well as on all nine subscales, with significant differences in seven of them. The differences were most profound on the subscales somatization and anger-hostility.

Table 9. SCL-90-R, Bern Embitterment Questionnaire, and IES-R scores

	Embittered (*n* = 49) Mean (SD)	Control Group (*n* = 50) Mean (SD)	*p* *t*-test
SCL global scores			
GSI	1.13(0.55)	0.74(0.50)	0.001***
PST	52.22(17.22)	39.30(19.49)	0.001***
PSDI	1.86(0.51)	1.57(0.41)	0.002**
SCL subscales			
Somatization	1.12(0.60)	0.69(0.54)	0.001***
Obsessive-compulsive	1.48(0.81)	1.08(0.80)	0.015*
Interpersonal sensitivity	0.95(0.74)	0.68(0.71)	0.063
Depression	1.55(0.74)	1.05(0.71)	0.001***
Anxiety	1.20(0.71)	0.76(0.68)	0.002**
Anger-hostility	0.97(0.63)	0.47(0.44)	0.001***
Phobic anxiety	0.67(0.55)	0.47(0.64)	0.104
Paranoid ideation	1.07(0.78)	0.60(0.58)	0.001***
Psychoticism	0.60(0.50)	0.36(0.36)	0.009**
Bern scale (*n* = 49/49)	2.29(0.68)	1.37(0.61)	0.001***
IES-R total score (*n* = 38/42)	3.12(0.81)	1.46(1.12)	0.001***
IES-R-Intrusion	3.68(0.89)	1.69(1.38)	0.001***
IES-R-Hyperarousal	3.38(0.94)	1.36(1.34)	0.001***
IES-R-Avoidance	2.42(1.12)	1.36(1.08)	0.001***

Note: * = p ≤ .05; ** = p ≤ .01; *** = p ≤ .001

Significantly higher scores for the PTED sample were also found for the IES-R and the Bern Embitterment questionnaire (IES-R total score = 3.12 vs. 1.46; Δ = 1.66; t (74.685) = -7.619, p < .001; Bern Embitterment questionnaire total score = 2.29 vs. 1.37; Δ = 0.92; t (96) = -6.994, p < .001). The PTED sample also scored significantly higher (p < .001) on all three subscales of the IES-R, i.e., intrusion, hyperarousal, and avoidance.

Conclusions on the psychopathology of PTED

The data show that patients with PTED are severely ill in respect to psychopathology. Results demonstrate that patients who react with prolonged and pathological embitterment to a negative life event can develop pronounced psychopathological symptoms. This shows that PTED must be considered not only as a "psychological problem" but as a severe type of illness. Clear differences between the PTED sample and the control group were found with regard to the quality and intensity of psychopathology as well as posttraumatic stress symptoms. These data show that patients with PTED can be discriminated from patients with other mental disorders.

Similar to anxiety or depression, embitterment must be understood as a dimensional phenomenon which becomes pathological when reaching greater intensities, when it is associated with additional symptoms, and when daily role performance is impaired. Our patients undoubtedly fulfill these criteria and must be called ill.

In contrast to adjustment disorders, the symptomatology found in PTED does not show a tendency towards spontaneous remission. On the contrary, patients tend to actively keep memories of the event alive.

Given the fact that 50% of our patients fulfill the criteria of major depression and 97.9% reported persistent negative mood, it might be argued that a majority of our patients had depression rather than PTED. It is well established that negative life events predict future depression (Kendler et al. 1999; Franko et al. 2004). Roberts et al. (1998) sees rumination, defined as a repetitive pattern of thoughts and behaviors that focus an individual's attention on their depressed state (Donaldson & Lam, 2004), as a vulnerability factor for depression. In addition, the psychopathological dimensions of anger, irritability, aggressiveness, and hostility in depression have recently received greater recognition in the literature (e.g., Pasquini et al. 2003; Benazzi 2003). However, despite overlaps with depressive symptoms, PTED is a distinct concept with its own symptomatology and etiology. In contrast to depression, affect modulation is unimpaired, as patients with PTED can display normal and positive affect when distracted or engaged in revenge fantasies. In depression, in contrast to PTED, the association between negative life events and depressive symptoms reflects not only a causal, but also a reciprocal relationship in which earlier depressive symptoms predict later negative events (Patton et al. 2003). In PTED, a negative life event is decisive for diagnosis (Linden et al. 2003). The symptomatology found in PTED, including aggressive tendencies, intrusive thoughts, and anger, can only be appropriately described and understood in connection to this specific event.

PTED and PTSD are similar disorders that are both characterized by a negative precipitating event, persistent psychopathological impairment and the characteristic symptoms of intrusion and numbness. They are different with respect to the type of precipitating event (life threatening vs. common life problem), the core psychopathology (anxiety vs. embitterment), and different treatment requirements.

The data show that PTED patients perceive the trigger event as traumatic. They determine the onset of their suffering to the day and hour, and they experience themselves as "being hurt" by the event, which is synonymous to being traumatized. This finding was also supported by the results of the IES-R, which revealed a high amount of posttraumatic stress among PTED patients, as well as an attentional focus towards the trigger event. From a clinical and scientific perspective, the term "trauma" also seems to be suitable because it emphasizes the specific connection between the trigger event and the psychopathological reaction. While in PTSD, fear of death and panic are specific etiological factors, PTED can be seen as a disorder in which the pathogenic properties of information are the decisive factors.

Finally, the differences between the groups on the Bern Embitterment questionnaire support the postulated central role of embitterment in PTED.

2.2 Diagnostic Interview and Criteria for PTED

Diagnostic criteria for PTED

The first patients were diagnosed according to clinical judgement. For further research, standardized diagnostic criteria and interviews are needed. Table 10 presents the clinical diagnostic criteria which summarize clinical experiences with these patients and specify their characteristic features.

Table 10. Clinical diagnostic criteria for PTED

Diagnostic Features
The essential feature of PTED is the development of clinically significant emotional or behavioral symptoms following a single exceptional, though normal negative life event. The person knows about the event and perceives it as the cause of illness. The event is experienced as unjust, as an insult, and as a humiliation. The individual's response to the event must involve feelings of embitterment, rage, and helplessness. The individual reacts with emotional arousal when reminded of the event. The characteristic symptoms resulting from the event are repeated intrusive memories and a persistent negative change in mental well-being. Affect modulation is unimpaired and normal affect can be observed if the individual is distracted.

The trigger event is a single negative life event that can occur in every life domain. The event is experienced as traumatic due to a violation of basic beliefs. Traumatic events of this type include, but are not limited to, conflict in the workplace, unemployment, death of a relative, divorce, severe illness, or experience of loss or separation. The illness develops in the direct context of the event. The person must not have had any obvious mental disorder prior to the event that could explain the abnormal reaction.

Associated Features
Individuals with PTED frequently manifest decreased performance in daily activities and roles. PTED is associated with impaired affectivity. Besides prolonged embitterment, individuals may display negative mood, irritability, restlessness, and resignation. Individuals may blame themselves for the event, for not having prevented it, or for not being able to cope with it. Patients may show a variety of unspecific somatic complaints, such as loss of appetite, sleep disturbance, pain.

Table 10. (continued)

Specific Culture Features
Elevated rates of PTED may occur in times of major social changes that force people to reorganize there personal biographies.

Differential Diagnosis
Despite partial overlaps in symptomatology, PTED can be differentiated from other affective disorders, PTSD, or anxiety disorders.

In contrast to *adjustment disorder* the symptomatology of PTED does not show a tendency towards spontaneous remission.

In contrast to *depression*, affect modulation is unimpaired in PTED. The specific causal connection between the trigger event and symptomatology found in PTED is not evident in depression.

While in *PTSD* anxiety is the predominant emotion, in PTED it is embitterment. In PTSD there must be a critical event that has to be exceptional and life threatening and that, most importantly, invariably leads to acute panic and extreme anxiety. In PTED there is always an acute event that can be called normal as it can happen to many people in a life course. Still, it is also an exceptional event as it is not an everyday event for the individual.

Diagnostic Criteria for PTED
A. Development of clinically significant emotional or behavioral symptoms following a single exceptional, though normal negative life event.
B. The traumatic event is experienced in the following ways:
   (1) The person knows about the event and sees it as the cause of illness.
   (2) The event is perceived as unjust, as an insult, and as a humiliation.
   (3) The person's response to the event involves feelings of embitterment, rage, and helplessness.
   (4) The person reacts with emotional arousal when reminded of the event.
C. Characteristic symptoms resulting from the event are repeated intrusive memories and a persistent negative change in mental well-being.
D. No obvious mental disorder that could explain the abnormal reaction was present prior to the event.
E. Performance in daily activities and roles is impaired.
F. Symptoms persist for more than 6 months.

These clinical criteria can be translated into research diagnostic criteria as summarized in Table 11. They have been developed by means of a comparison between PTED and control patients. In section A, three criteria are given that must all be fulfilled. Of the five further symptoms listed in section B, four must be answered with yes. The duration should be longer than six months and there should be no other mental disorder which could explain the onset of the illness.

Table 11. Research diagnostic criteria for PTED

Section A: All questions must be answered with yes.		
A1: During the last years, was there a severe event/experience that hurt your feelings and caused considerable embitterment?	Yes	No
A2: Did this event lead to a noticeable and persistent negative change in your mental well-being?	Yes	No
A3: Do you experience the critical life event as unjust? Do you have the feeling that destiny or the responsible person has treated you unfairly?	Yes	No
Section B: Four questions must be answered with yes.		
B1: During the last months, did you have repeatedly intrusive and incriminating thoughts about the event?	Yes	No
B2: Does it still extremely upset you when you are reminded of the event?	Yes	No
B3: Does the critical event or its originator make you fell helpless and disempowered?	Yes	No
B4: Is your prevailing mood since the critical event frequently down?	Yes	No
B5: If you are distracted, are you able to experience a normal mood?	Yes	No
Section C: Duration must exceed six months.		
C1: For how long have you already been suffering from psychological impairment caused by the event? (Specify in months.)	Longer than 6 months	
Section D: No other disorder can explain the present mental state.		
D1: Prior to the event, did you suffer from any (substantial/relevant/noticeable) psychological or mental problems (depression, anxieties or the like)?	Yes	No

Development of a semi-structured diagnostic interview

These research diagnostic criteria can be assessed by a semi-standardized diagnostic interview for PTED (see Appendix). At the beginning of the interview, each patient is asked whether they have, during the last years, experienced an event that considerably hurt their feelings. Since one can expect that insulting experiences are a frequent condition in everyday life, and the patient may have experienced more then one hurtful event during the last years, the interview structure gives the patient the chance to record more than one negative event on a list. The assessment of multiple events enables the researcher to explore possible additive effects (Strain et al. 1999) of critical events. After this general recall of critical events, the patient is asked to determine the one event that is most important for his or her present mental state. The patient is asked whether this event was the cause of a persistent negative change in his or her mental well-being, and whether any psychological or mental problems was present prior to the event. Then the core characteristics of PTED, the emotional spectrum patients experience when reminded of the event, and psychopathological signs and symptoms are explored. In order to capture the specific connection between the critical life event and the psychological response, which is postulated in the concept of PTED, the questions of the interview are all asked in reference to the event.

Applying a semi-standardized interview meets the methodological requirements of life events research (see Paykel, 1983; Paykel, 2001a; Petermann, 1995). A semi-structured interview with some probing and flexibility is seen as the method of choice for the collection of life events data (Paykel, 1983; Paykel, 2001a).

The discriminatory power of the interview and of each item was analyzed, and a diagnostic algorithm which allowed the best differentiation of both groups was derived. The item combination of the semi-standardized diagnostic interview that allows the best differentiation of both groups (i.e., with reference to sensitivity and specificity) is presented in Table 11. All questions of Section A need to be answered with yes. At least four of the questions in Section B need to be answered with yes, and the duration of illness (Section C) needs to be longer than 6 months. If there were any relevant psychological or mental problems prior to the event (Section D), no diagnosis of PTED can be made.

On the basis of this diagnostic algorithm, 47 of the 50 PTED patients were diagnosed as having PTED, thus the sensitivity was 94%. Four patients of the 50 control group patients, who had been classified as non-PTED patients by a clinician, were diagnosed as having PTED on the basis of the diagnostic algorithm. Thus, the specificity was 92%.

In order to find the reasons for the conflicting classifications, the files of the respective seven patients were analyzed in more detail.

(1) The first inconsistently classified patient of the PTED sample was hospitalized due to inability to work. During the clinical interview, the patient reported a work-related incident as the cause of her impairment. Unjustified reproaches of evasions against her, and subsequent threats of dismissal were experienced as unjust, and as an insult. The patient reported feelings of embitterment, helplessness, and rage when thinking about the event. Based on clinical estimation and impression, the patient was diagnosed as suffering from PTED. However, the diagnostic algorithm classified the patient as not suffering from PTED as the patient denied that the critical event had led to a noticeable and persistent negative change in her well-being. The results of the self-report measures Bern Embitterment Questionnaire (Mean Total 1.70), the PTED self-rating scale[11] (PTED Scale; MT 2.29), and the IES-R (MT 2.64) revealed that an embitterment affect, PTED symptomatology, and posttraumatic stress were present in the patient. However, on all three scales the patient scored lower than the overall average of the PTED sample (Bern Embitterment Questionnaire/PTED Scale/IES-R: 2.29/2.64 /3.12).

(2) The second inconsistently classified patient of the PTED sample reported that he had suffered from psychological problems prior to the event, and was therefore classified as not suffering from PTED on the basis of the diagnostic algorithm. During the clinical interview the patient reported a number of critical events that were all job related. The first relevant event happened in 1996, when the patient was bullied at work by his boss, which had the consequence that the patient quit. This event was a traumatic experience for the patient as he had had close ties to his boss, and he felt like losing his "father figure". The patient reacted to this event with a workplace phobia, rumination, and psychosomatic symptoms (sick leave for six months). When he started a new job, further negative events occurred. The patient reported constant workplace bullying by his colleagues. Then an accident happened while at work, and finally the patient lost his job. This recent experience of losing his job was reported during the standardized assessment as the most important critical event for his present state. In the standardized interview, the psychological problems that occurred as a consequence of the first event (bullying by the boss in 1996) were coded as a preexisting mental disorder, and the patient therefore classified as not suffering from PTED.

In this case, one can assume that a diagnosis of PTED would be correct. During therapy, the patient reported that the recent negative event of losing his job reactivated the feelings which he experienced when he quit his job in 1996. In addition, he reported that he was still angry with his boss. Furthermore, the patient showed strong basic beliefs concerning honesty and justice, which

---

[11] The PTED Scale is a newly developed instrument to measure symptom severity in PTED. The PTED Scale will be introduced and discussed in chapter 2.3.

were challenged by the events. Moreover, above average scores (for the PTED sample) in the self-report measures Bern Embitterment Questionnaire (MT 3.40), the PTED Scale (MT 3.82) and the IES-R (MT 4.09) demonstrated that an embitterment affect, PTED symptomatology, and posttraumatic stress were present in the patient.

(3) The third inconsistently classified patient of the PTED sample lost her job due to illness (chronic pain in the back). During the clinical interview, the patient reported her unemployment to be the cause of indignation, embitterment, and anger. She felt like a "beggar." Still, in the standardized interview, she denied that this event had led to a noticeable and persistent negative change in her well-being. Thus the patient was classified as not suffering from PTED. The results of the self-report measures Bern Embitterment Questionnaire (MT 1.15), the PTED Scale (MT 0) and the IES-R (MT 0) support this classification. Moreover, no signs of reactive embitterment surfaced during treatment.

(4) The first patient of the control group who was inconsistently classified was hospitalized due to work incapacity. During standardized assessment, a critical life event (conflict in the workplace) was reported, and the following answers indicated severe PTED symptomatology. No psychological or mental problems prior to the event were reported. The results of the self-report measures Bern Embitterment Questionnaire (MT 1.35), the PTED Scale (MT 2.65) and the IES-R (MT 3.68) showed that an embitterment affect, PTED symptomatology, and posttraumatic stress were present in the patient. However, longitudinal evaluation and treatment of the patient revealed an agoraphobia which had persisted for 20 years. The presence of a mental disorder prior to the event does not allow a diagnosis of PTED.

(5) The second inconsistently classified patient of the control group did not show any signs of reactive embitterment during the clinical interview. He reported a discharge from his job as a critical event, but expressed relief rather than distress in connection to this event. The results of the self-report measures Bern Embitterment Questionnaire (MT 1.25), the PTED Scale (MT 1.65) and the IES-R (MT 1.86) support the classification of non-PTED. During the standardized assessment, though, the patient reported distress and psychopathological symptomatology in connection with the critical event.

(6) The third inconsistently classified patient of the control group reported bereavement (death of his son) as a critical life event during the clinical interview. The patient did not react with embitterment to this event, he rather showed normal mourning. The standardized assessment did not differentiate well enough between these two emotions. In the future, interviewers must be better trained to look at this problem.

(7) The fourth patient of the control group who was classified inconsistently denied the occurrence of any critical event during the clinical interview. In

contradiction to this statement, a critical event ("son abandoned his child") was reported during the standardized assessment. In addition, a great negative impact of this event on mental well-being was reported by the patient. The results of the self-report measures Bern Embitterment Questionnaire (MT 1.45), the PTED Scale (MT 1.47) and the IES-R (MT 3.59) indicate moderate embitterment and PTED symptomatology, and high posttraumatic stress. However, the examination of the patient's file did not reveal any more signs of a connection between the critical event and symptomatology. The critical event was not mentioned by the patient during psychotherapeutic treatment.

Standardized diagnostic interview for PTED

The analysis of the inconsistently classified patients revealed some shortcomings of the first version of the diagnostic interview. It is important for a diagnosis of PTED that the pre-morbidity of the patient is examined thoroughly, in order to rule out those patients who suffered from psychological or mental problems prior to the event. Patients with mental disorders can show a tendency to report critical events in order to give meaning and explanation to an illness. By doing this, the impact of an event is often overemphasized. For PTED, it is required that there is a connection between the critical event and the resulting psychopathology. Symptoms of PTED must not be explained by any preexisting psychological problems. Therefore, the exclusion of possible other reasons for illness onset is essential for a diagnosis of PTED.

In addition, the emotional quality of the reaction to a critical event must be specified. There are many possible emotional reactions to negative life events, and embitterment is only one. In order to rule out other reactive emotions, for example bereavement, one needs to assess the characteristic facets of embitterment. The results of the standardized diagnostic interview for PTED indicated that feelings of embitterment, rage, and helplessness (Items No. 12f, 12c, & 12h) in connection with the event are characteristic for patients with PTED. This emotional spectrum needs to be assessed in order to confirm embitterment as a reaction to a negative life event.

Another important aspect in the diagnostic process is the role of cumulative events in PTED. A recent minor life event superimposed on a previous major life event that has no observable effect on its own may have a cataclysmic effect due to its additive impact (Strain et al. 1999). Hence, the identification of the trigger event can be problematic. The critical event reported during the diagnostic interview may not be the trigger event, but the most recently experienced negative event. Thus, symptomatology prior to the reported event can

appear as a preexisting mental disorder, even though it occurred in response
to the actual trigger event.

These considerations were the basis for a refined version of the diagnostic
interview which is presented in Table 12. It thoroughly investigates the emotional
quality experienced in connection with the event. The interviewer is urged to
judge whether reactive embitterment is present or not. Subsequently, the clinician needs to assess whether any premorbid mental disorder could explain the
present psychopathology.

Table 12. The diagnostic interview for PTED

A. Core Criteria		
1. During the last years, was there a severe event/experi-ence that led to a noticeable and persistent negative change in your mental well-being?	→ NO	YES
2. Did you experience the critical life event as unjust or unfair?	→ NO	YES
3. Do you feel embitterment, rage, and helplessness when reminded of the event?	→ NO	YES
4. Did you suffer from any (substantial/relevant/notice-able) psychological or mental problems (depression, anxieties or the like) prior to the event?	NO	→ YES
EVALUATION BY THE EXAMINER:		
EMOTIONAL EMBITTERMENT (MARKED BY EMBITTERMENT, RAGE, AND HELPLESSNESS)?	→ NO	YES
CAN ANY PREMORBID MENTAL DISORDER EXPLAIN THE PRESENT PSYCHOPATHOLOGY?	NO	→ YES
5. For how long have you already suffered from psychological impair-ment caused by the event? (Specify in months.)		
_____ Months	→ Less than 6 months	

Table 12. (continued)

B. Additional Symptoms		
1. During the last months, did you repeatedly have intrusive and incriminating thoughts about the event?	NO	YES
2. Does it still extremely upset you when you are reminded of the event?	NO	YES
3. Does the critical event or its originator make you feel helpless and disempowered?	NO	YES
4. Is your prevailing mood since the critical event frequently down?	NO	YES
5. If you are distracted, are you able to experience a normal mood?	NO	YES
ARE FOUR QUESTIONS IN SECTION B ANSWERED WITH YES?	$\rightarrow$ NO	YES
POSTTRAUMATIC EMBITTERMENT DISORDER	NO	YES

Note. The Answers marked with an arrow indicate that one of the essential criteria for the diagnosis of PTED is not met. Thus, the clinician is asked to directly indicate "NO" in the diagnostic box at the bottom of the interview.

The diagnostic criteria for PTED, which were established on the grounds of clinical experience with these patients and empirical data from clinically defined PTED patients and patients with other mental disorders, show that PTED can be diagnosed objectively. For research purposes, a semi-standardized interview can be used to assess the core criteria. It is essential to note that not the event itself but the psychopathological reaction defines PTED. Being betrayed by your spouse or being humiliated at work is not an illness. Showing prolonged embitterment after such an event, with impairment in activities of daily living, suicidal ideation, sleep disorders, repetitive intrusive thoughts, irritability, loss of appetite, lack of drive, etc. defines an illness state which can be summarized as PTED and discriminated from other mental disorders.

2.3 The PTED Self-Rating Scale

In addition to the diagnostic interview for PTED, an instrument is needed to quantify the emotional reaction in PTED. Embitterment is a natural emotional reaction to an insult. Thus, embitterment must be understood as a dimensional phenomenon that only becomes pathological when reaching greater intensities. A method of assessing symptom severity in PTED can be the self-rating of the patient.

For this purpose, the PTED Self-Rating Scale (PTED Scale) was developed, an instrument which can be used to measure symptom severity in cases of PTED. The PTED Scale can also serve as a screening instrument.

The following sections describe the PTED Scale and data on the reliability, validity, internal consistency, test-retest reliability; a principal component analysis and data on convergent and discriminant validity are also presented.

Construction of the PTED Self-Rating Scale

The PTED Scale is a 19-item questionnaire designed to assess the diagnostic criteria of PTED (see Appendix). The characteristic features of PTED were summarized and translated into self-rating questions. The questionnaire starts with the instruction "Please read the following statements and indicate to what degree they apply to you." In order to capture the specific connection between the critical life event and the psychological response which is characteristic for PTED, each question starts with the line "During the last years there was a severe and negative life event...," which is then followed by statements such as "...that hurt my feelings and caused considerable embitterment." For each item, patients are asked to indicate to what extent the statement applies to them on a 5-point Likert scale. The scale comprises the values (0) "not true at all," (1) "hardly true," (2) "partially true," (3) "very much true," to (4) "extremely true."

The PTED Scale was administered to two samples: (1) Seehof sample: Consisting of a PTED sample and a control group (see the section on the psychopathology of PTED above). Due to missing data, 4 subjects were excluded from the analyses, which resulted in an overall sample size of $N = 96$, with $n = 48$ for each group. (2) Unselected inpatients (UI): 100 randomly selected inpatients (73 women, 27 men) from the Psychosomatic Rehabilitation Hospital Heinrich Heine, Potsdam, Germany, which provides treatment for patients who suffer from all kinds of chronic mental disorders. The age of patients ranged from 27 to 63 years (Mean = 46.9; $SD = 8.76$). 76% of the participants lived in a permanent relationship (74% were married), 24% lived alone. 80% of the participants had one or more children. The highest formal education level reached was elementary or basic secondary school level[12] for 59% of the patients, 30% had finished high school.[13] 72% had a permanent occupation, 19% were unemployed. In this sample, the scale was administered twice with a time interval of 6–8 days.

During these studies, which took place over a time span of 2 years, the scale was slightly changed in order to remove some lack of clarity. Two items of the original 17-item scale were split into two items each, which resulted in the 19-item scale. The Seehof sample was assessed with the 17-item version, the 19-item version was utilized in the UI sample.

Reliability

The ratings of the UI sample on all items of the PTED Scale are given in Figure 4 (first assessment) in descending order. The alpha coefficient was .93, indicating a high internal consistency. The test-retest reliability (time interval of 6–8 days) of the PTED Scale was assessed using the Spearman Rho correlation as a coefficient, which measures associations at the ordinal level. Due to missing data (more than 13% missing answers, i.e., 5 out of 38 items), 5 participants were excluded from the analyses (Wirtz, 2004). As indicated in Table 13, the correlations between the two time points were high, ranging from .53 to .86, with all reaching significant levels ($p \leq .01$). A mean total correlation of .71 indicates a high reliability over time.

Principal component analyses

A principal component analysis was calculated on all PTED Scale items using data of the UI sample. The number of factors to be extracted was determined according to the scree-plot method (Cattell, 1966). Two factors emerged, accounting for 55.25% of the total variance. After orthogonal rotation using the varimax technique, a simple structure was obtained (see Table 13). All variables were well defined by this factor solution, as indicated by moderately high communality values (Range = 0.33–0.79). Factor I was defined by items that ask for psychological status and social functioning. Factor II was defined by items that ask for emotional responses to the event, and for thoughts of revenge. This

---

[12] German: Hauptschule
[13] German: Abitur (qualifies for university entrance)

Figure 4. Frequency distribution of the unselected inpatient sample for each item of the PTED Scale (*N* = 100)

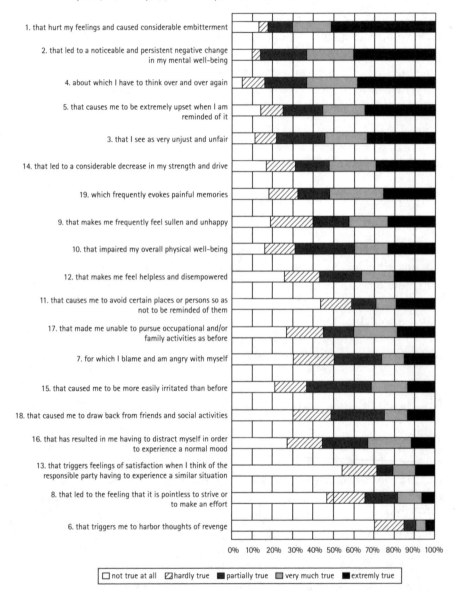

In the last years (about 3-4 years) I had to cope with a harmful life event ...

1. that hurt my feelings and caused considerable embitterment

2. that led to a noticeable and persistent negative change in my mental well-being

4. about which I have to think over and over again

5. that causes me to be extremely upset when I am reminded of it

3. that I see as very unjust and unfair

14. that led to a considerable decrease in my strength and drive

19. which frequently evokes painful memories

9. that makes me frequently feel sullen and unhappy

10. that impaired my overall physical well-being

12. that makes me feel helpless and disempowered

11. that causes me to avoid certain places or persons so as not to be reminded of them

17. that made me unable to pursue occupational and/or family activities as before

7. for which I blame and am angry with myself

15. that caused me to be more easily irritated than before

18. that caused me to draw back from friends and social activities

16. that has resulted in me having to distract myself in order to experience a normal mood

13. that triggers feelings of satisfaction when I think of the responsible party having to experience a similar situation

8. that led to the feeling that it is pointless to strive or to make an effort

6. that triggers me to harbor thoughts of revenge

0% 10% 20% 30% 40% 50% 60% 70% 80% 90% 100%

□ not true at all   ▨ hardly true   ■ partially true   ▨ very much true   ■ extremly true

Table 13. Spearman Rho Coefficients (time interval of 6–8 days), rotated
factor solution and within-group correlations with the discriminant
function.

PTED Scale items	Spear-man Rho Coefficients	Factor I	Factor II	Within-group correlations with the discriminant function
1. that hurt my feelings and caused considerable embitterment	.640**		0.55	.643
2. that led to a noticeable and persistent negative change in my mental well-being	.706**	0.74		.599
3. that I see as very unjust and unfair	.716**		0.70	.671
4. about which I have to think over and over again	.742**	0.60		.689*
5. that causes me to be extremely upset when I am reminded of it	.713**	0.58		.745
6. that triggers me to harbor thoughts of revenge	.540**		0.70	.435*
7. for which I blame and am angry with myself	.620**		0.62	.380
8. that led to the feeling that it is pointless to strive or to make an effort	.663**	0.52		.689
9. that makes me frequently feel sullen and unhappy	.819**	0.84		.699
10. that impaired my overall physical well-being	.753**	0.80		.622

Table 13. (continued)

11. that causes me to avoid certain places or persons so as not to be reminded of them	.796**	0.49		.500
12. that makes me feel help-less and disempowered	.726**	0.67		.693
13. that triggers feelings of satisfaction when I think of the responsible party having to experience a similar situation	.537**		0.57	.435*
14. that led to a considerable decrease in my strength and drive	.783**	0.89		.593
15. that caused me to be more easily irritated than before	.681**	0.75		.669
16. that has resulted in me having to distract myself in order to experience a normal	.775**	0.84		.653
17. that made me unable to pursue occupational and/or family activities as before	.742**	0.81		.588
18. that caused me to draw back from friends and social activities	.722**	0.62		.347
19. which frequently evokes painful memories	.867**	0.79		.689*
Mean Total:	.713**	Variance explained: 39.19%	16.06%	

Note. ** Significance level $p \leq .01$.
       The Spearman Rho Coefficients and the factor analysis were carried out
       using data of the UI sample.
       The discriminant function was calculated using data of the Seehof sample.
* The within-group correlations with the discriminant function were obtained from
a 17-items version of the PTED Scale. In this version, items 6 & 13 and 19 & 4
were summed up in one item. The coefficients marked with an asterisk are obtained by these summed up versions of the respective items.

factor solution comprises two core dimensions of psychopathology in PTED: a) The pathological emotional reaction following a negative life event, and b) the resulting impairment of mental well-being and social functioning. Therefore, it appears appropriate to use a total score of the PTED Scale in order to evaluate the severity of PTED symptomatology.

Validity

The validity of the PTED Scale was assessed by means of a discriminant analysis using the PTED sample and the matched control group (Seehof sample). In this analysis, the 17-item version of the PTED Scale was utilized. The mean scores of the subsamples of the Seehof sample on each item are illustrated in Figure 5. Patients with PTED showed significantly higher scores on the PTED self-report questionnaire with a mean total of 2.64 (SD = .93) for the PTED sample, and 0.92 (SD = .77) for the control group (t (94) = -9.84, p < .001. Significant (p < .001) differences were also found for each item of the questionnaire.

A χ^2 transformation of Wilks' lambda indicated that the computed discriminant function discriminated significantly (χ^2 = 76.51, p < .001) between the two groups. Forty-three of the 48 PTED patients were diagnosed as having PTED on the basis of the PTED Scale, thus the sensitivity was 89.6%. Four of the 48 control group patients who had been classified as non-PTED patients by a clinician were diagnosed as having PTED on the basis of the PTED Scale. Thus, the specificity was 91.7%. Overall, the predicted classification based on the PTED Scale was in accordance with the clinical diagnoses in 90.6% of all cases.

The discriminant function indicated a mean total cut-off score of 1.6, suggesting that subjects who score an average of 1.6 or more on the PTED Scale suffer from prolonged embitterment with an intensity of clinical relevance. With regard to clinical practicability, and in order to increase specificity, a mean total cut-off score of 2 is suggested.

Table 13 shows the within-group correlations with the discriminant function for each item. Moderate to high correlations were found for each item, indicating that all items are of discriminant value. Particularly high correlations were found for items asking for intrusive memories (items 4, 5, and 19), for feelings of disempowerment, helplessness and injustice (items 1, 3, 8, and 12), and for items concerning deterioration of mood and numbness (items 9, 15, and 16). These findings reflect three characteristic features of PTED symptomatology:

a) the central role of a negative life event which frequently triggers painful and intrusive memories,

b) the feeling of helplessness and injustice caused by the event, and

c) the resulting deterioration of mental well-being.

Figure 5. Mean scores of both subsamples of the Seehof sample for each item of the PTED Scale (*N* = 96, 17-item version)

In the last years (about 3–4 years) I had to cope with a harmful life event ...

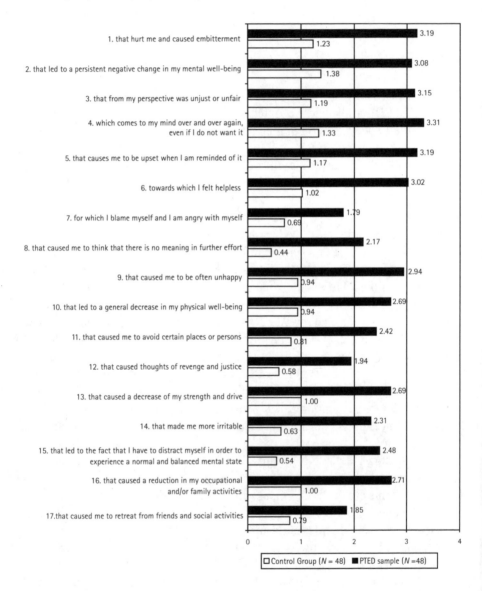

□ Control Group (*N* = 48)   ■ PTED sample (*N* =48)

Convergent validity

The convergent validity was assessed using data of the PTED sample. Table 14 presents the relationships between the scores obtained from the PTED Scale, the IES-R, the SCL-90-R, and the Bern Embitterment Questionnaire. As expected, significant correlations ($p < .001$) were observed between PTED scores and measures of embitterment, posttraumatic stress, and psychopathological symptoms.

Table 14. Intercorrelations of the PTED Scale with concurrent validity measures assessed with data from the PTED sample ($n = 48$)

Measure	1	2	3	4	5	6
1. PTED- Scale	–					
2. IES-R Total	.76	–				
3. Bern Embitterment Questionnaire	.67	.53	–			
4. SCL- GSI	.57	.55	.60	–		
5. SCL- PST	.52	.56	.56	.90	–	
6. SCL-PSDI	.49	.46	.56	.83	.57	–

Note: $p < .001$ for all correlations.
PTED Scale = PTED Self-Rating Scale; IES-R = Impact of Event Scale-Revision; SCL = Symptom Checklist 90 Revised; GSI = Global Severity Index; PST = Positive Symptom Total; PSDI = Positive Symptom Distress Index.

The data show that the PTED Scale is an instrument which can be used to measure symptom severity in cases of PTED, similar to anxiety scales for anxiety disorders and depression scales for depressive disorders. Furthermore, the PTED Scale can serve as a screening instrument to alert physicians to PTED symptomatology. The PTED Scale is a reliable and valid measure for embitterment as an emotional reaction to a negative life event. The Scale can, to some extent, even distinguish between those with and without PTED. A mean total score ≥ 2 on the PTED Scale indicates a clinically significant intensity of reactive embitterment. The internal consistency and the retest reliability were relatively high. The construct validity of the PTED Scale was demonstrated by the high concordance (90.6%) with clinical diagnoses. Convergent validity could be shown as there were significant correlations with the Bern Embitterment Questionnaire, the IES-R, and the SCL-90-R.

2.4 The Epidemiology of PTED

PTED is a prototypical reaction type to negative life events that violate basic beliefs. One can expect that such experiences and events are frequent in everyday life and that PTED therefore can be seen at all times and in all places (Linden, 2003). Increased numbers can be expected under social conditions that force significant numbers of individuals to cope with fundamental changes in their job situation and in their families, as it was seen after the German reunification (Linden, 2004). The question is what the base rate is in the general population or in specific groups of patients. To get initial epidemiological data on PTED, the PTED Self-Rating Scale was administered to several samples drawn from different populations.

Reactive embitterment in a train sample

158 passengers travelling on trains from Berlin to Frankfurt/Oder between 7:00 am and 8:00 pm on weekdays were asked to fill in the PTED Self Rating Scale. In order to enhance representativity of the sample, equal distribution was aimed for on 2 (gender) × 5 (age-group) factor levels. Instructions were given in a standardized manner, and each participant was informed about study procedures, data protection, and the participant's right to terminate participation at any time. All participants signed an informed consent form in which they declared that they had been informed about the purposes of the study and were willing to participate.

29.5% of the participants were university graduates and 62.2% were in full-time employment. 65.2% were married and 19.6% lived in a long-term partnership. Table 15 summarizes the socio-demographic data of the train sample and illustrates the distribution of women and men for the different socio-demographic categories.

On average, 67.5% of the participants indicated that the statements of the PTED Scale did not apply to them at all. The percentages for the answer category 0 ("not true at all") ranged from 44.1% for item 1 ("...that hurt my feelings and caused considerable embitterment"), to 87% for item 15 ("...that has resulted in me having distract myself in order to experience a normal mood"). 17% of the participants showed some tendency to agree with the statements ("hardly true"). 8.7% specified that the statements partially applied to them ("partially true"), and 3.4% of the sample indicated that they agreed with the 17 items ("very much true"). An average of 3.3% reported that the statements totally applied to them

Table 15. Sociodemographic data of the train sample for women and men
        (*N* = 158)

	Men *N* = 73	**Women** *N* = 85	**Total** *N* = **158**
Age			
20–29 years	10.8%	12.7%	23.4%
30–39 years	7.0%	8.9%	15.8%
40–49 years	8.9%	13.3%	22.2%
50–59 years	9.5%	9.5%	19.0%
60–65 years	10.1%	9.5%	19.6%
Education level			
Non-university graduate	32.7%	37.8%	70.5%
University graduate	13.5%	16.0%	29.5%
Occupational situation			
Full-time employment	30.1%	32.1%	62.2%
Trainee	4.5%	9.6%	14.1%
Retired	7.7%	10.9%	18.6%
Not working	3.2%	1.9%	5.1%
Family status			
Long-term single	1.3%	5.7%	7.0%
Short-term single	1.9%	3.8%	5.7%
Changing partnerships	1.3%	1.3%	2.5%
Long-term partnership	9.5%	10.1%	19.6%
Married	32.3%	32.9%	65.2%

("extremely true"). The percentages for the answer category 4 ("extremely true") ranged from 0% for item 8 ("…that led to the feeling that it is pointless to strive or to make an effort") and item 13 ("…that led to a considerable decrease in my strength and drive") to 9.9% for item 3 ("…that I see as very unjust and unfair"). The highest scores were obtained for items 1 and 3, with an average score >1. The lowest ratings were found for items 10 and 15 (average score = .23/.21).

Looking at the item-specific results in more detail, 34.8% of the participants indicated that they had experienced an event that hurt their feelings and caused considerable embitterment (item 1).[14] 35.4% had experienced the critical event as unjust and unfair (item 3) and 27.9% reported repetitive painful memories of the event (item 4). 14.8% indicated that the negative life event had led to a noticeable persistent negative change in their mental well-being (item 2). 22.3% reported that remembrance of the event caused them to be extremely upset (item 5). Moreover, 22.9% felt helpless and disempowered because of the event. Figure 6 illustrates the frequency distribution for the different answer categories for each item.

Figure 6. Frequency distribution (in %) of the train sample (*N* = 158) for the five-point answer categories of each item on the PTED Scale

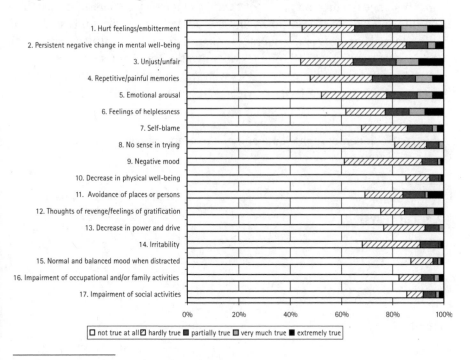

<hr>

14 The three answer categories "partially true," "very much true," and "extremely true" are here and in the following interpreted as an (at least partial) affirmation of the respective item.

A mean total score of .58 (*SD* = .60; Range = 0–2.76) was obtained. Four participants (2.5%) showed a mean total score higher than 2, indicating a clinically significant intensity of reactive embitterment (see chapter 2.3.). 43 participants (27.2%) with a mean total score of 0 did not show any signs of reactive embitterment. Taking a mean total score of 1 as an indication of the presence of reactive embitterment, it can be assumed that embitterment in connection to a negative life event is known to 25.3% of the train sample.

Reactive embitterment in patients of general practitioners

221 patients of three general practitioners (GP sample) were asked to fill in the PTED Self-Rating Scale. Ninety-nine patients were recruited in a practice in Berlin-Charlottenburg, and 56 patients in a practice in Berlin-Wilmersdorf, two western districts of Berlin, and 66 in Gnoien, a village in the eastern part of Germany.

Every patient in the waiting room was asked to participate. All participants were informed about study procedures, data protection, and the participant's right to terminate participation at any time. Following this introduction, participants signed an informed consent form in which they declared that they had been informed about the purposes and the procedures of the study and were willing to participate. As the average time a patient has to wait in a general practice is approximately 48 minutes, there was no time pressure.

71.5% (*n* = 158) of the participants were women and 28.5% men (*n* = 63). Age ranged from 15 to 81 years (Mean = 42.5; *SD* = 13.8). The majority of

Table 16. Sociodemographic data and occupational situation of the GP sample (*N* = 221)

	General physician patients
Age (in years)	
Range	15–81
M	42.5
SD	13.8
Gender	
Female	158 (71.5%)
Male	63 (28.5%)

Table 16. (continued)

Family status	
Unmarried	84 (38%)
Married	97 (43.9%)
Divorced	28 (12.7%)
Widowed	12 (5.4%)
Origin	
Former East Germany	66 (29.9%)
Former West Germany	155 (70.1%)
Highest level of school education completed	
No formal school education	2 (0.9%)
Special needs education	2 (0.9%)
Elementary or secondary school level 1	132 (59.7%)
High school	80 (36.2%)
Miscellaneous	5 (2.3%)
Current occupation	
Full-time employed	68 (30.8%)
Part-time employed	29 (13.1%)
In vocational training	30 (13.6%)
Unemployed	44 (19.9%)
Retired	14 (6.3%)
Time-limited retirement due to work incapacity	5 (2.3%)
Unlimited retirement due to work incapacity	11 (5%)
Professional development	3 (1.4%)
Other	17 (7.7%)

participants were married (43.9%), 38% were unmarried, 12.7% divorced, and 5.4% widowed. 64.3% of the participants had children. 23.5% of the participants had finished college or university. 70.1% of the sample lived in urban regions (Berlin) and came from the former West Germany. 29.9% lived in a rural area. All subjects from the rural area came from the former East Germany. Table 16 gives an overview of socio-demographic data and the present occupational situation of participants.

On average, 10.4% of the participants indicated that all 19 items of the scale totally applied to them ("extremely true"). The percentages for the answer category "extremely true" ranged from 23.1% for item 1 ("…that hurt my feelings and caused considerable embitterment") to 2.3% for item 8 ("… that led to the feeling that it is pointless to strive or to make an effort"). 13.6% of the participants indicated that the 19 statements applied to them ("very much true"), and 14.4% specified that the statements partially applied to them ("partially true"). Another 14% of the sample showed some tendency to agree with the statements ("hardly true"). Moreover, about 50% (maximum 70.6%) said that the statements of the PTED Scale did not apply to them ("not true at all").

Looking at the item-specific results in more detail, about 61.1% of the participants indicated that they had experienced a life event that hurt their feelings and caused embitterment (item 1). An equal number of participants reported repetitive memories about the event (item 4). 37.6% saw the event as very unjust and unfair, and another 12.2% experienced the event as partially unjust and unfair (item 3). 53.8% were upset when reminded of the event (item 5), and the event frequently evoked painful memories in 51.6% of the participants (item 19). 29.8% indicated that the negative life event led to a noticeable persistent negative change in their mental well-being, and for 16.7% this was partially true (item 2). 19.4% reported that the event led to an impairment of their overall physical well-being, and 14% indicated a partial impairment (item 10).

Items that referred to thoughts of revenge (item 6 and 13), avoidance behavior (item 11), and strive inhibition and inhibition of social and family/occupational activities (items 8, 17, and 18) showed the lowest scores overall. Figure 7 illustrates the frequency distribution for the different answer categories for each item.

Looking at the embitterment symptoms in more detail, repetitive memories and emotional arousal when reminded of the event seem to play a prominent role. Nearly all participants who reported an event that triggered embitterment also reported that they had to think about the event over and over again. About half of these participants suffered from emotional arousal when reminded of the event, feelings of injustice, and a persistent negative change in their psychological well-being.

Figure 7. Frequency distribution (in %) of the GP sample (*N* = 221) for the five-point answer categories of each item on the PTED Scale

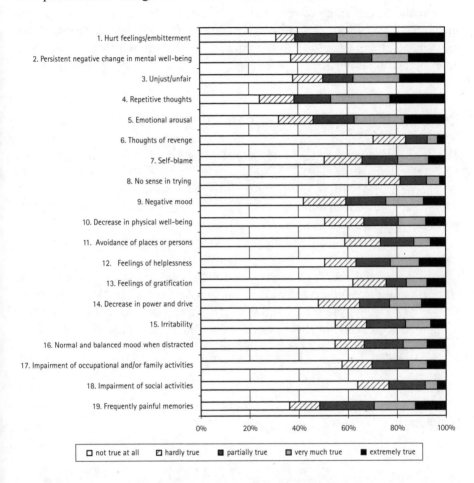

Thoughts of revenge, drive inhibition, and impairment of social activities seem to play a subordinate role in reactive embitterment. However, the low rating of the revenge item could be explained by the fact that this emotion is not well accepted socially. Thus participants may tend to conceal this emotion.

A mean total score of 1.22 (*SD* = .94; range = 0–3.68) was obtained. Fifty-three participants (24%) showed a mean total score higher than 2, indicating a clinically significant intensity of reactive embitterment (see chapter 2.3). Twenty-seven participants (12.2%) did not show any signs of reactive embitterment (mean total score = 0). Taking a mean total score of ≥ 1 as an indication of the presence of reactive embitterment, it may be assumed that embitterment is known to 55.2% of the GP sample. However, one needs to consider that all participants filled in the self-report questionnaire while waiting for an appointment with their general practitioner. Hence, it can be assumed that most of the participants did not feel well at the time of assessment, which may have had an exaggerating influence on the results.

Comparison of clinical and non–clinical samples

The distributions of the mean total scores of the four different samples on the PTED Scale are illustrated in Figure 8.

There are clear differences in the distribution of mean total scores between the four samples. Mean total was 2.64 (SD = .93; range = 0–3.88) for the PTED sample, 1.95 (SD = .92; range = 0–3.89) for the UI sample, 1.22 (SD = .94; range = 0–3.68) for the GP sample, and .58 (SD = .60; range = 0–2.76) for the train sample.

The mean total scores showed approximately normal distribution in both clinical samples, as indicated by the Kolmogorof-Smirnov test (PTED sample: Z = .71, p = .70; UI sample: Z = .80 p = .55). In the non-clinical samples, the mean total scores did not show a normal distribution (GP sample: Z = 1.46, p = .028; train sample: Z = 2.06, p < .001)

Figure 8. Frequency distributions of four different samples on the PTED Scale (mean total scores)

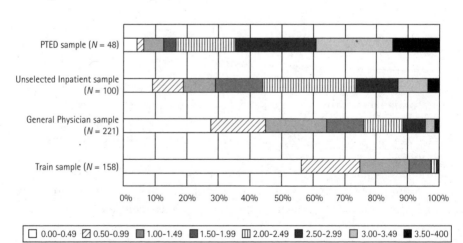

The results of these first epidemiological studies show that embitterment as a reaction to a negative life event is a prevalent phenomenon among clinical and nonclinical populations. Reactive embitterment is an emotion which is known to about 25% of the general population, as can be assumed from the train sample (mean total score ≥ 1). About one third reported that they had experienced a severe and negative event during the last years, which hurt their feelings and caused embitterment. Equal numbers reported a persistent negative change in their mental well-being as a direct consequence of the event. However, only 2–3% of the train sample were suffering from PTED symptoms to a degree which undoubtedly must be called a state of mental disorder (mean total score > 2). In this respect, embitterment must be understood as a dimensional phenomenon similar to anxiety or deterioration of mood. Increasing intensity leads to a change in quality. In comparison to other mental disorders, the estimated prevalence rate of 2–3% indicates that PTED is a mental disorder with an epidemiologically relevant magnitude.

These findings were supported by the examination of patients of general physicians. In comparison to the train sample, the occurrence and the intensity of embitterment symptoms were higher in the GP sample. About 60% reported a critical event that triggered embitterment. In addition, 46.5% reported a persistent negative change in their mental well-being. Embitterment of clinically significant intensity was indicated by 24% of the GP sample. These findings emphasize the importance of acknowledging the impact of single exceptional, though normal negative life events. The development of clinically relevant symptoms in the direct context of such an event seems to be frequent among patients of general physicians.

The results of the UI sample, with 53% of the patients showing a mean total score ≥ 2, suggests that reactive embitterment plays a prominent role among inpatients with mental disorders. One can assume, given the results of the UI and GP sample, that some cases which are presently diagnosed as depression or phobia are in fact cases of PTED.

Overall, the epidemiological data presented in this chapter supports the assumption that embitterment is a common reaction to negative events that can be seen at all times in all places (Linden, 2003). The results of the PTED Scale revealed that reactive embitterment and associated symptoms are prevalent in clinical and nonclinical populations, and can occur in different intensities until the point of clinical relevance.

However, the PTED Scale is not sufficient to establish a diagnosis of PTED, thus it can only serve as a screening instrument in such populations. Therefore, the results presented in this chapter can only indicate whether characteristic symptoms of PTED are present or not. A diagnosis of PTED can only be made on the basis of a thoroughly assessment of the patient. Thus nothing can be said about the actual presence of the syndrome on basis of the PTED Scale alone. However, considering the results presented in this chapter, it can be assumed that an undiagnosed base rate of PTED is present in clinical and nonclinical populations.

2.5 Wisdom and Activation of Wisdom-Related Knowledge in PTED

Assessment of wisdom

In order to empirically validate the assumption that patients with PTED display a deficiency in activating wisdom-related knowledge when confronted with difficult life problems, wisdom-related performance in PTED patients was assessed. This was done in 49 PTED and 49 control patients (see Chapter 2.1.). In accordance with the work of Baltes & Smith, (1990), Baltes & Staudinger (2000), and Böhmig-Krumhaar et al. (2002) the method of irresolvable problems was used to assess wisdom-related performance. All participants were confronted with fictitious unsolvable life problems under standardized conditions, such as the following example:

'Mr. Smith has been accused of fraud and has been imprisoned for six months. When innocence is proven, he is discharged. Meanwhile his wife has left him'.

The participants were then asked to discuss aloud what came to their mind if they thought of Mr. Smith. They were asked what they would do. Eight problems of this type were used in the present study. All of them were negative life events, involving three people, and none had a clear solution. Wisdom-related knowledge was also assessed in respect to personal life problems. Participants were asked how they had so far tried to cope with life events that led to their inpatient treatment. Responses were recorded on tape and transcribed. Subsequently, three trained clinicians evaluated the protocols of the respondents in light of nine wisdom-related criteria (see Chapter 1.5), using a five-point scale ranging from "not at all" (0) to "very much" (4).

Training of wisdom-related knowledge

PTED and control patients were additionally subdivided into an intervention and a nonintervention group (two PTED/control intervention groups, $n = 24$; and two PTED/control nonintervention groups, $n = 25$). For both intervention groups, two sessions of wisdom training were administered in which participants were given more fictitious life problems. Participants were stimulated to comment on these in a structured way. They were asked to describe, comment on, and solve the life problems from different perspectives and in reference to different persons, contexts, and value systems. They were, for example, asked what a grandmother would say and do, who had managed to get her children through the war and had mastered a lot of difficulties in her life, or a manager who is a rational person and engaged in practical problem-solving, or a priest who is engaged in moral and philosophical questions, or a psychologist who deals with human behavior and problems, or an anthropologist who is engaged in studying the way of life, culture, and habits of people in Africa.

After the training was completed, all participants were reassessed for wisdom-related performance. The time period between the two assessments (pre-/posttest) ranged from 1 to 9 days. However, because Böhmig-Krumhaar, Staudinger, and Baltes (2002) found a negative retest effect in wisdom-related tasks, which they explained by an exhaustion-effect and motivation decrease, we followed their suggestion and used different life-problems at each point of assessment to decrease retest-effects. Furthermore, the nonintervention groups allow to compare retest-effects with the intervention effect.

Wisdom in PTED patients and patients with other mental disorders

PTED patients showed an overall lower wisdom-related performance in relation to fictitious life problems than patients from the control group (Mean total score = 1.56 vs. 2.07; $\Delta = 0.51$; $t_{89.12} = 3.26$, p = .002). They also scored lower on all nine wisdom scales, with significant differences on 7 of them (change of perspective: $t_{96} = 2.26$, p = .026; acceptance of emotions: $t_{83} = 2.85$, $p = .005$; serenity: $t_{95} = 2.06$, $p = .042$; factual knowledge: $t_{96} = 3.37$, $p = .001$; contextualism: $t_{95} = 2.22$, $p = .029$; uncertainty acceptance: $t_{82.83} = 2.47$, $p = .016$; long-term perspective: $t_{96} = 3.69, p < .001$). The items empathy ($p = .062$) and value relativism ($p = .088$) did not show significant differences between groups. The lowest scores for the PTED sample were obtained for the wisdom criteria long-term perspective, uncertainty acceptance, and change of perspective. Figure 9 illustrates the wisdom-related performances of both groups in connection to fictitious life problems.

No differences were found between the intervention and nonintervention groups in the pretest assessment.

The PTED sample also showed lower scores than the control group in relation to the personal problem in the pretest (Mean total score = 1.16 vs. 2.05; $\Delta = 0.89$; $t(84.92) = 6.25, p < .001$). Moreover, with the exception of acceptance of emotions, significant differences were found on all subscales ($p < .001$). In contrast to the fictitious problem condition, the PTED sample showed noticeably lower scores in the personal problem condition (MT = 1.16 vs. 1.56; $\Delta = .40$). This was not observed in the control group, which showed similar scores in

Figure 9. Wisdom-related performance of the PTED sample and the control group ($N = 98$) in connection to fictitious life problems on the nine wisdom scales (pretest assessment)

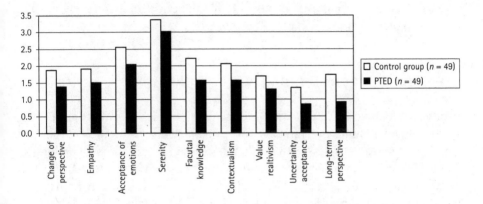

Missing data: PTED sample ($n = 42$) for acceptance of emotions. Control group ($n = 48$) for serenity, contextualism, uncertainty acceptance; $n = 43$ for acceptance of emotions.

Figure 10. Wisdom-related performance of the PTED sample and the control group ($N = 98$) in connection to a personal life problem on the nine wisdom scales (pretest assessment)

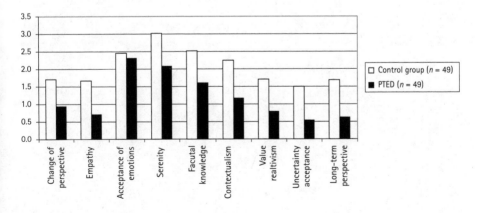

Missing data: PTED sample ($n = 48$) for serenity, factual knowledge, contextualism, value relativism, uncertainty acceptance, long-term perspective; $n = 41$ for acceptance of emotions. Control group ($n = 43$) for acceptance of emotions.

both conditions (MT = 2.05 vs. 2.07; Δ = .02). The lowest scores for the PTED sample were obtained for the wisdom criteria long-term perspective, uncertainty acceptance, and empathy. Figure 10 illustrates wisdom-related performance of both groups in connection to personal life problems.

Again, no significant differences were found between the intervention and nonintervention group in the pretest assessment.

Effects of wisdom training

In order to examine the intervention effects, a one-way analysis of variance and a set of planned multiple comparisons were calculated for wisdom-related performance in the posttest assessment in relation to fictitious and personal problems. Table 17 shows the linear nonorthogonal contrasts between intervention and nonintervention groups and PTED and control patients. It was hypothesized that both intervention subsamples would show higher wisdom-related scores in the posttest assessment than the nonintervention subsamples. Furthermore, it was assumed that the trained PTED patients would show equal wisdom scores in the posttest assessment as the patients of the control group. In order to account for the nonorthogonality of the contrasts tested, a Bonferroni-adjusted alpha level was used (α_{PC} = .05/c = .013), resulting in a familywise error rate $(1-(1- \alpha_{PC})^4)$ of α_{FC} = .05.[15]

Table 17. Set of linear nonorthogonal contrasts

Contrasts	Factor Levels			
	Control group/ no training	Control group/ training	PTED sample/ training	PTED sample/ no training
1.	0	0	1	-1
2.	1	-1	0	0
3.	1	1	-2	0
4.	1	1	0	-2

---

[15] Abbreviations: α_{PC} = per comparison error rate; α_{FC} = familywise error rate; c = number of comparisons.

Figure 11. Mean total scores of each group for the pre- and posttest in the fictitious problem condition

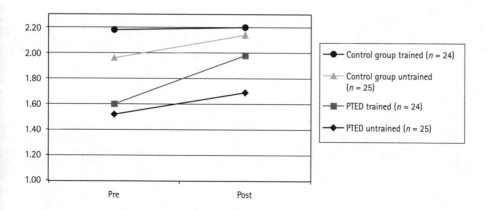

Missing data: Control group untrained (n = 24) and PTED trained (*n* = 23) in posttest assessment.

Figure 11 illustrates the mean total scores of each group for the pre- and posttest in the fictitious problem condition.

The PTED patients that received wisdom training showed the biggest increase in overall wisdom-related performance in connection to a fictitious problem (pre-/posttest: 1.6/1.98). However, the untrained PTED patients also showed higher wisdom scores in the posttest, suggesting that factors other than the intervention accounted partially for the observed increase in wisdom-related performance.

In contrast to the trained control group patients, the untrained control patients showed an increase in wisdom-related performance in the posttest assessment (pre-/posttest: 1.96/2.14), indicating that no intervention effects where present in the trained control group.

No significant differences between the groups in the posttest assessment were found for wisdom-related performance in connection to fictitious problems (F (3, 91) = 2.06, p = .111). In addition, none of the four contrasts reached significant levels, indicating that the intervention did not lead to an increase in wisdom-related performance. However, contrast number 4 just missed significant levels (t (92) = 2.463, p = .016), suggesting that mainly the increase in performance in the trained PTED subsample led to the observed equalization of wisdom scores between PTED sample and control group in the posttest assessment.

Figure 12 illustrates the mean total scores of each group for the pre- and posttest in the personal problem condition.

Figure 12. Mean total scores of each group for the pre- and posttest in the personal problem condition

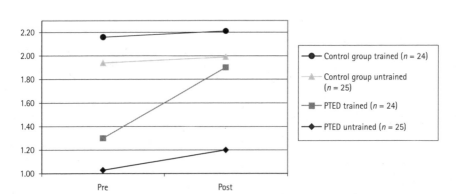

Missing data: Control group untrained (*n* = 24) and PTED trained (*n* = 22) in posttest assessment.

As in the fictitious condition, the trained PTED patients showed the biggest increase in overall wisdom-related performance in connection to a personal problem (pre-/posttest: 1.3/1.87). The overall wisdom scores of the untrained PTED subsample increased only slightly (pre-/posttest: 1.03/1.18). Thus, one can assume that the observed increase in wisdom-related performance in trained PTED patients resulted from the training program.

No change in wisdom-related performance in connection to a personal problem was observed in either subsample of the control group in the posttest assessment.

Significant differences between the different groups were indicated for wisdom-related performance in the posttest assessment (F (3, 91) = 10.23, *p* < .001). The multiple comparisons revealed significant differences between the subsamples of the PTED sample (Contrast No. 1: *t* (35.855) = 4.315, *p* < .001), and between the untrained PTED patients and the control group (Contrast No. 4: *t* (68.268) = 6.319, *p* < .001). No differences were found between the control group subsamples (Contrast No. 2: *t* (44.28) = .959, *p* = .343), and between the control group and the trained PTED patients (Contrast No. 3: *t* (49.35) = 1.17, *p* = .249).

Figure 13 illustrates the wisdom scores in connection to a personal problem on all nine wisdom scales for the subsamples of the PTED sample in the post-test assessment.

Figure 13. Wisdom-related performance of the subsamples of the PTED
sample in connection to a personal life problem on the nine wisdom scales
(posttest assessment)

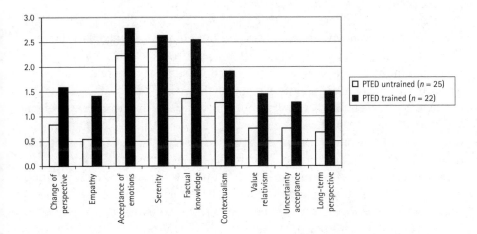

Missing data: PTED trained (*n* = 18) for acceptance of emotions; *n* = 21 for uncertainty
acceptance. PTED untrained (*n* = 22) for acceptance of emotions; *n* = 24 for value
relativism.

The trained PTED patients scored higher on all nine wisdom scales in the
personal problem condition than the untrained PTED patients. Significant differences were indicated for 8 of them (change of perspective: $t(44) = -2.81, p =$
.007; empathy: $t(44) = -3.28, p = .002$; acceptance of emotions: $t(38) = -2.14$,
$p = .039$; factual knowledge: $t(45) = -6.21, p < .001$; contextualism: $t(45) =$
$-3.16, p = .003$; value relativism: $t(45) = -2.82, p = .007$; uncertainty acceptance:
$t(34.71) = -2.13, p = .041$; long-term perspective: $t(32.6) = -2.60, p = .014$;).
Scores on the item serenity did not show significant differences ($p = .314$).

Conclusion

Clear differences in regard to wisdom-related performance were found between
PTED patients and patients with other mental disorders. Patients with PTED
showed significantly lower wisdom scores in connection to fictitious as well as
to personal life problems. These findings empirically support the assumption
that patients with PTED show a deficiency in activating wisdom-related knowledge systems when confronted with difficult life problems. This deficiency is
particularly prominent in connection to the trigger event (personal condition).

PTED patients seem to lack the ability to activate knowledge systems that could enable them to cope with the experienced insult. In particular, they seem to be unable to accept uncertainty, to show empathy, and to apply a long-term perspective when confronted with the trigger event.

In contrast to the personal condition, relatively high wisdom scores were found in connection with fictitious general life problems in the PTED sample (MT = 1.16 vs. 1.56; Δ = .40). These differences across the two conditions were not found in the control group. Thus, one can assume that there is no general deficiency in activating wisdom-related knowledge in PTED. Rather, a specific deficiency can be observed, which is probably caused by the disorder and which impairs the application of wisdom resources specifically in connection with the trigger event. This implies that the therapeutic task is to help patients with PTED to activate their wisdom knowledge in respect to their personal problem.

Moreover, our study demonstrates that a relatively short training program can activate wisdom-related knowledge in PTED. No differences in wisdom were found in posttest assessment between the PTED training subsample and the control group. In the personal condition, this equalization of wisdom scores can clearly be attributed to the training program. In the fictitious condition, the training program can only partly account for the increase in wisdom scores. A possible explanation for the absence of a training effect in the fictitious condition is the relatively high level of performance at pretest assessment. The high scores may have left only little room for progress.

While the training program proved to be useful for patients with PTED, no intervention effects were found in the control group. Whether this is caused by a ceiling effect cannot be decided on the basis of the present data.

Overall, the empirical findings on wisdom and the activation of wisdom-related knowledge in PTED suggest that cognitive interventions aiming at wisdom enhancement could prove effective in treating PTED.

3. Treatment Perspectives

3.1 Cognitive Behavior Therapy for PTED

General treatment perspectives

The therapy of chronic adjustment disorders and PTED can pose considerable problems. Particularly the core emotion of embitterment can lead to a rejection of treatment. Patients want the world to see how bad they have been treated, and they often do not seek treatment on their own. Our own patients regularly came after their health insurance asked them to seek inpatient treatment because of prolonged sick leave. Furthermore, therapy is often complicated by a fatalistic-aggressive attitude of the patients, which obstructs the process of developing new life perspectives, and new perspectives on what happened to them (Schippan, Baumann, & Linden, 2004). There is at present no consensus treatment for PTED.

Patients who have experienced a traumatic life event need to emotionally reprocess the emotional insult and debasement. The helplessness experienced and the agitation of basic beliefs about the world and oneself need to be processed in order to establish an inner distance to the event, as well as the possibility to develop new life perspectives (Schippan et al. 2004).

Procedures of this type have been described in the context of logotherapy by Frankl (1998) who has, amongst others, worked with survivors of the Holocaust. Logotherapy aims at giving a new meaning in a larger context to negative events. This can be understood as a reframing procedure changing not only the cognitive but also the emotional meaning of the critical event. This is embedded in a stepwise process as it has been described in the context of abnormal grief, ranging from denial via anger and despair to, finally, acceptance. Humanistic psychology and client-centered psychotherapy (Tausch, 1992) have also pointed to the importance of forgiving, if self-destructive embitterment is really to be overcome.

Whether exposure techniques such as used in PTSD (Maercker, Böhmig-Krumhaar, Staudinger, 1998) will also be of help in PTED is an open question. These techniques work in PTSD when patients learn response control. In PTED it is hypothesized that patients will only benefit from exposure if it enables them to change their views on the meaning of the event.

From a psychobiological point of view, the task must be to support the cortical integration of trauma memories into general semantic networks, thus reducing the strength of hippocampally mediated and emotionally laden memories of the insult (Stickgold, 2002; Gottschalk, Fronezek, Abel, Buchsbaum, Fallon, 2001).

Cognitive–behavioral treatment for PTED

Patients with PTED must learn how to cope with negative life events and to solve life problems. These are traditional treatment goals in behavior therapy. There are numerous methods of how to help patients with such problems. Inflexibility of basic beliefs is thought to be another important aspect in PTED. There are also many established techniques in cognitive behavior therapy, which aim at modifying cognitions and attitudes and which therefore can also be used in PTED (Linden, 2003). Still, as discussed before, there are special problems in using such conventional methods in PTED patients, as they react differently than many other patients, especially being not very cooperative. Therefore, special adaptations of such classic interventions are needed. Based on the theoretical considerations about the etiology of PTED, on the available empirical findings, and on clinical experience, Schippan et al. (2004) developed a treatment approach especially for PTED. In the following, this newly developed treatment approach that accounts for specific characteristics of PTED will be discussed in more detail.

Therapeutic relationship

The first therapeutic task is to develop a working relationship between therapist and embittered patient. Patients with PTED are often distrustful and fatalistic, reacting cynically and reproachfully against themselves and against the therapist and rejecting treatment and offers of help. Therefore, special therapeutic efforts are necessary to establish a trustful and cooperative patient-therapist relationship.

Initially it is important to avoid the impression that the patient is seeing the therapist in order to change. Patients interpret any idea that they should change as an implicit suggestion that they themselves are responsible for what happened. They see the aggressor as responsible and therefore the aggressor and the outer world must do something to achieve reconciliation, not the patient. Therefore, the patient should be granted a "time-out". That is, it should be made clear that nobody wants the patient to change, or to do anything.

The therapist is there only to listen and understand and empathize with the patients and their feelings. Even more, the therapist is a person who might help to find justice. It is important to understand the point of view of the patient. Appreciation of the patient's suffering and clear judgments about the injustice that has occurred are needed so that the patient does not get the feeling that he or she has to justify his or her view again. PTED initially demands a lot of empathy, and unconditional acceptance by the clinician. One therapeutic method that can be used are reflective verbalizations and the repetition of judgments as made by the patient: "I understand that one is hurt when such a thing happens, this has been really unjust, etc."

Analysis of the critical life event, associated emotions, and basic beliefs

Only once the patient feels that the therapist is on their side and sees "what has happened" can the patient's central motives, values, and basic beliefs, which have been violated and called into question be assessed. In this treatment phase, the clinician must stay on the patient's side without any ifs and buts. This treatment phase begins by asking the patient to tell "more" about the critical event. The clinician should explicitly point out that they understand that recalling the event can be stressful and disturbing. The patient tends to give global appraisals. The therapist wants to know more and therefore asks for details in a descriptive way, which adds objective data on what happened. Who did what, how, and when?

The patient is not only asked to say what happened but, even more, how they felt. The patient is stimulated to give their "evaluations" in the form of feelings and emotions. Patients with PTED tend to disclaim negative and undesirable emotions. Especially, "unacceptable" emotions like anger, humiliation, and thoughts of revenge are often denied and suppressed by the patient because they contradict their self-concept or moral beliefs. It can be helpful to enforce negative emotions by empathic feedback. The therapeutic method is to summarize emotions of the patient as emotions which are held by the therapist ("If my wife did this, I could beat her; when I hear what you say, thoughts of revenge come to my mind, I would throw stones at his car").

After behavior and emotions, cognitions must also be assessed. The therapist asks for the subjective experiences, perceptions, and evaluations of the patient in connection with the event: "What is it, that hurt you most? What made you really mad?" PTED is not triggered by the critical life event as such, but by the violation of basic beliefs and values. Therefore the question is what caused the humiliation, the feelings of injustice, and the personal insult. The aim is to identify the basic beliefs and values that were decisive for the development of the disorder.

Assessment of intrusions, avoidance behavior, and changes in everyday life

The next step is to analyze what the critical event and the embitterment have done to the patient. There is the problem of intrusive thoughts. As the memories of what has happened are emotionally laden they come to the patient's mind over and over again. It can be helpful to ask the patient to observe and count how often per hour they are reminded of or think about what has happened. Patients must observe and learn that bad memories lead to bad emotions, and that they feel bad whenever they are reminded of the critical event. The question to the patient is whether they can stop thinking. If these are intrusive thoughts, they cannot be stopped.

There is the further problem of avoidance. Stimuli like company logos, post-boxes, or children in the street can remind patients of their humiliation over and over again. Patients tend to avoid such places or persons. They do no longer shop in certain shops or even avoid going to certain areas of the city as this reminds them of what has happened or presents the danger of meeting somebody who has been involved in what happened. Places, persons, or situations that could remind patients of the event are often avoided because exposure leads to a decrease and avoidance to an increase in their subjective well-being. Patients do not identify their behavior as avoidance behavior. Instead, they talk about having "no inter-est" or that they "do not feel like it", or do not "want" to go to such places. In the end it is important for patients to realize that avoidance behavior is not under their control but an element of the disorder. Only by carefully asking for such behavior will the extent of this self-inflicted impairment become obvious.

Closely associated with avoidance is impairment in everyday living. Patients retreat from friends and even from their family. They no longer attend social or cultural events. They do not feel like this. Their whole life can change dramati-cally. Participation in all areas of life is reduced or threatened. Embitterment results in avoidance of the workplace and colleagues, in social withdrawal, problems in the partnership, or in abandoning hobbies and interests. All life domains need to be scrutinized for such secondary problems.

Introduction of an illness concept and encouragement of treatment motivation

Patients with PTED initially tend to make one-sided allocations of guilt, and to revel in grudges and cultivate their anger ("The world should see how badly I have been treated!"). They remain passive in cynical devaluation ("If life is not just, then nothing has any sense!"; "Why should I try to change something, if others play pranks on me?"). If this attitude is not overcome, every further treatment is doomed to failure.

While the patient came initially with the idea that "the" problem is what happened, they now learn that they are not only punished by the critical event but even more by the consequences of their present state of mind. There is a double punishment. The question is: "How come that you allow the aggressor to punish you twice, first by the critical event and now by social withdrawal and bad mood?"

Even though patients deny that they suffer from an illness, they do feel very bad. With empathy and sympathy it is possible to communicate to the patient that they do not deserve this, and that they have suffered enough, and how wonderful it would be, if they could again freely look forward and leave the past behind. Patients do not understand their embitterment as morbid. It is rather seen as an unpleasant feeling justified by external reality, and hence appropriate. It can be helpful to point out that there are other patients with similar experiences ("Your story reminds me of ...; I often encounter cases like yours..."). Clarification and description of the full range of symptoms can help the patient to realize that the critical event is a problem but that the persistent emotional consequences are a problem as well. By telling the patient that their reaction is experienced by other patients in the same way, embitterment is made a "normal" and a pathological reaction at the same time. As it is no longer in the hand of the patient to free themselves from this state of mind, professional help could be a way out. At this point the patient can become motivated not to change his views of what has happened but to change his present state.

Activation of resources, increase of activities, and paradoxical interventions

A first way of reactivating the patient is to capitalize on the "double-punishment" idea. As a consequence, a paradoxical intervention can be used. The aggressor is "punished" by not allowing him to influence one's life. "Well-being" can become a form of revenge: "My boss shall regret whom he has fired! I won't let the aggressor destroy my life! I do not allow the aggressor to prevent me from going to the cinema! I will punish my husband by dressing up and making other men look at me!" Another idea is that "well-being" is a necessary prerequisite to better fight with the aggressor: "I will lose in court, if I am in bad shape!" Also, thoughts of "justice" can be helpful. "After all they did to me I deserve compensation." Patients regularly voice this thought themselves. They want a pension "as compensation." The therapeutic suggestion is that somebody who has suffered deserves to get something good and that doing good things for oneself and caring about oneself can also be a form of satisfaction.

The patient is not able to change the critical event, but they are able to influence the continuing consequences. The question is what their coping repertoire looks like. How has the patient tackled life problems in the past? The focus is on the patient's expertise and coping resources. Patients with PTED have often been quite successful in their life. Therefore, they possess many abilities. Embitterment prevents them from using these and doing what they can. This is similar to depression and other pathological emotional states. The same is true for social resources. Are there friends and family members who are on the side of the patient? If one wants to stand up, one needs allies.

There is also the question of feelings of guilt towards the beloved ones: "Do I allow the aggressor to also inflict harm on my wife, as in my present state I am no longer a good and caring husband?" Patients are asked to discriminate between friend and foe. Embitterment and aggression must become discriminate: "Be nice to friends and harsh to enemies!"

Exposition

Embittered patients show phobic avoidance of persons and places that remind them of the critical event. As in anxiety disorders, this avoidance behavior shows a tendency to generalization, and can lead to total withdrawal. Similar to the treatment of anxiety disorders or PTSD, a systematic exposition for the reduction of avoidance behavior can be helpful in treating PTED. Patients are asked to interact with their environment again. They are asked to go out into public, to go back to their workplace, and to fight the constriction of their social and professional life. Helpful cognitions can be: "I do not need to hide!," "I won't break!," "I will go through this standing tall," "To go through this standing tall is the biggest achievement of my life!" and so forth. In this vein, paradox intervention can again be helpful ("I punish the aggressor by confronting him upright and proud").

New perspectives

The critical life event often leads to significant changes in life perspective and life planning (e.g., by unemployment, illness, or separation). Thus, one aspect of therapy needs to be the development of alternative perspectives, which counteract the development of additional embitterment. In this connection, the clinician needs to take into consideration the basic beliefs and values that guide the patient, and which have been called into question by the critical event. In many cases it is necessary to integrate new life goals and new interpretations of life into the life planning. New life goals with an "inner" meaning are more likely to be valued as a new start by the patient. Short- and long-term plans that are realistic and appropriate for the patient and possible alternatives should be outlined explicitly.

3.2 Wisdom Therapy

Expertise to cope with unsolvable life problems

The core problem in PTED are violations of basic beliefs. All the beforementioned interventions did not touch on the question why the critical event was humiliating. Instead, this was taken as given. Still, in order to overcome PTED, it is necessary to (re)process the experienced humiliation and the insult, and to reach an inner reconciliation with the event and the originator. The patient needs to bring the past to a close, and built up new life perspectives for the future. In order to do this, the activation of wisdom can be helpful.

The inflexibility of basic beliefs as found in PTED can best be described by referring to modern wisdom psychology (Erikson, 1976; Baltes & Smith, 1990; Staudinger & Baltes, 1996a; Staudinger, Lopez, Baltes, 1997). In reference to the Berlin wisdom paradigm (Baltes & Staudinger, 2000), Schippan et al. (2004) developed "wisdom therapy" as a new treatment approach specifically designed for PTED. Based on wisdom psychology, special interventions were developed to enhance change of perspectives, distancing of oneself, empathy, acceptance of emotions, serenity, sense of humor, factual knowledge, contextualism, value relativism, self-relativization, uncertainty acceptance, long-term perspective, reevaluation of problems and goals. The therapy for PTED tries to activate and enhance wisdom-related knowledge and strategies. A specific therapeutic intervention is the method of irresolvable problems. A prerequisite for the application of this intervention is that the patient is, through the previous treatment steps, ready and capable of thinking, in conjunction with the clinician, about possible solutions to and alternative perspectives on their problem.

Factual knowledge and long-term perspective

Many patients try to find the reasons that caused the critical life problem, in order to solve it. They are guided by the dysfunctional assumption that knowledge of the causes would bring a solution. Others try to reverse the consequences of the event. They are determined to fight, even in hopeless situations. A patient may not want to stop even after losing their case in the high court, wanting to start all over, start new court cases, "talk" again with the former employer, or apply to the president of the state.

The question which the patient has to answer is: What are the realistic options and the remaining possible action when looking at the problem not from an emotional but a rational perspective. What are the "facts"? Is further information needed? Where can one get reliable information on what is possible? When will I ask whom what? The patient should be stimulated to describe and recognize effective and ineffective strategies.

In doing that, the question arises what effectiveness means. The opponent is dead or also humiliated? I get my job back? Does "effectiveness" refer to emotional satisfaction or factual solutions? What is effectiveness in a short-term or long-term perspective? This can help to solve the contradiction between the current need for revenge and the long-ranging want for limitation of damage. Therapeutic methods are, e.g., time projection: "Imagine you are ten years older than today. What is the advantage of living during the next ten years with or without a man who cannot fully be trusted?"

Acceptance of emotions and emotional serenity

When looking at the event and possible solutions from an emotional and a rational view, a split in perspectives arises. The patient gets the subjective feeling of having "two hearts in his chest." One that will fight on, whatever the cost, and another that wants to forget and go on. The emotion is stronger. Therefore, the question is how to get control over the embitterment. Once again, the full blend of emotions, and especially "unacceptable" emotions (e.g., anger after a husband has committed suicide, thoughts of revenge after having lost a job, humiliation because somebody else was promoted) should also be described and accepted as given. A therapeutic method can be cognitive rehearsal, i.e., vividly reminding oneself of all details and looking at the accompanying emotions. The therapist can help with this emotional clarification by reflecting and summarizing what they see and hear while the patient is rehearsing what has happened.

To accept the presence of emotions can help to feel no longer angry, irritated, and overwhelmed by one's emotions. There are special therapeutic interventions to further emotional serenity. A first step is self-monitoring and an early awareness of emerging negative emotions, in order to counteract emotional flooding. The patient can practice looking at his/her emotions from a metaperspective ("Now I am going to get angry!") in order to gain control. Negative emotions often indicate a threat to one's own plans and goals. Thus, it can be helpful to identify these threatened plans, and to analyze whether the arising negative emotions can save them, or if there is something else one could do. Also, distraction can be helpful or taking a time-out and leaving the present situation for a moment. Another cognitive strategy is to build up a rivalry over the control of the patient's emotions between the patient and the "offender".

This can be established by, for example, asking the patient how much power over their feelings and emotions they want to give to the "offender".

In summary, this phase of treatment can be characterized by a shift from *"embitterment" is the appropriate evaluation of the critical event* to *embitterment has become a problem of its own and must be brought under control.*

Change of perspective

One possibility to change emotions is to reevaluate what has happened. It is natural that somebody who was let down takes a personal and one-sided view on the events. But, this must include distorted perceptions and recollections of what happened, i.e., further increase the humiliation. Therefore it is helpful to look at what happened from the perspective of the aggressor. What made him act as he did? Would I have acted differently, if I had been in his position? The patient is asked to put themselves into the place of the "offender", and to empathize with their motives and emotions. This opens the opportunity to recognize that the "offender" may have acted in reaction to practical constraints. Hence, their actions may have had legitimate origins, and do not necessarily constitute a personal attack or devaluation (e.g., after occupational transfer or dismissal). In doing so, the patient regains psychological control over the events.

However, the understanding of different behaviors as a result of different roles is not the only goal, but also the experience and perception of typical emotions of the "other side." In this connection, the patient is asked to imagine emotions of the "offender" in a concrete and differentiated way. Here the clinician should pay attention that the patient does not only ascribe negative emotions to the "offender." It may be helpful to introduce a differentiation between the "offender" as a carrier of a role (e.g., boss), and as a private person. This differentiation allows the imagination of ambivalent and contradicting emotions.

Contextualism and value relativism

Value relativism and contextualism are important abilities that help to distance oneself from the irreversibility of one's own conclusions and judgments. Many PTED patients unchangeably adhere to their ideas of justice, honor, innocence, and guilt. They must learn to see that this is relative. The landlord has a different perspective and evaluation of how high a reasonable rent should be than the tenant; the employer takes other factors into consideration than the employee. Role changes beyond the persons directly involved can be helpful to accept that justice can mean different things to different people and that one's own perspective is valid but that one cannot expect everybody to share this view.

Similarly, a "change of situation" can be helpful. The same life problem (e.g., losing one's job) has different meanings in different places. A certain sum of money after a divorce may not be "enough" in one's own perspective, but could still be a lot of money for many other people. This helps to put one's own evaluations in a larger context and find more "objective" frames of reference in judging what is right and wrong.

Acceptance of uncertainty and powerlessness

One problem is that patients fear the critical event could come back again in the future: "The next husband will leave me as well, the other child could die as well, a new job will be endangered as well." The same is true in cases where the future development is still at stake, e.g., after a divorce, in problems with children, or after being given a new position at work. Patients must learn to accept uncertainty as a normal and integral part of life. In other cases the problem is that there is no chance to make the critical event undone or reverse its consequences, e.g., the suicide of a husband. In many patients, both feelings of uncertainty and powerlessness lead to feelings of unbearable helplessness. Patients have to learn that fighting is good when you can win and get control over events but that acceptance of the inevitable is also a very important and valuable human capacity.

In this regard re-attribution strategies can be helpful. Even though they cannot reduce the material damage, they can lead to an intellectual or emotional gain. This can be discussed with the patient on a metalevel, or one of the following perspectives can be brought up. In doing this, the therapist should refer to the biography and personality of the patient. Depending on the patient's basic beliefs and views of the world, they can be asked what the experience can teach them. The critical event can be seen as a test (by God or life) that needs to be accomplished. Only in rough waters can the captain show what he is worth. Only sorrow makes life worth living, because only where sorrow is joy can be as well. Humility, i.e., the insight into necessity and the will to accept the circumstances, can be seen as competency or virtue. The notion that people who overcome difficult life problems have a high social reputation can be helpful.

Another approach is to change the focus of attention. Patients focus on what they lost. This presents an obstacle to seeing what they have and what can still be done. Attention must be directed to the remaining options. The blocking of old goals is always a chance for a new beginning. One can start to look for advantages, chances, and options (chance for a new beginning; interruption of the "boring" normal course of life) that come about through the critical event.

The method of unsolvable problems

Experience with embittered patients has shown that, even after comprehensive preparatory work, they are often not able to establish sufficient distance to their own situation to recognize new ways of confronting their problem. They frequently fall back into old reasoning and reaction patterns. Therefore, the method of irresolvable problems was developed. In this method, patients learn to activate wisdom-related knowledge and wisdom-related strategies to cope with difficult life problems through guided reflection about a fictitious problems. This knowledge can later be adopted when confronted with their personal problems. The work on fictitious problems reduces the risk of adverse reactions by patients, as they are not personally concerned, and no "correct" solutions are forwarded by the therapist. Instead, different solutions are possible in regard to different contexts.

The helplessness of the patient in regard to their ability to solve difficult life problems is a good starting point for talking about basic principles of how to cope with critical life events. Thus, a general "problem solving training" is initiated. Ways of coping with life crises and disappointments are gathered in regard to a fictitious life problem. In doing so, strategies of looking at a problem from different perspectives, of developing empathy for the counterpart, of establishing distance to oneself, of integrating contradicting cognitive and emotional aspects into the solution and conclusions are practiced. Furthermore, openness for new experiences is developed, and the willingness to confront difficult problems in a differentiated way by considering different reference systems and metaaspects is activated. The required wisdom skills are described and summarized in the course of the training, by referring to individuals generally seen as "wise." Rather incidentally, the stepwise transfer of the acquired skills onto personal problems can take place.

Table 18 lists fictitious life problems that can be utilized in wisdom therapy. All dilemmas are ill-defined, profoundly negative life events with more than one person concerned and without a clear solution. All training problems are short descriptions of unjust and difficult, yet common events that are mostly irreversible and can cause embitterment. The descriptions deliberately leave room for speculation and interpretation. It is advisable to start the training with a problem that differs from the personal problem of the patient (e.g., a relationship conflict, if the patient's embitterment is caused by conflicts at the workplace). Thereby, it is possible to first practice problem-solving strategies in connection to dilemmas that do not concern the patient personally. Further training-problems, even though they should differ from the patient's personal problem, can take place in the same problem domain.

Table 18. List of fictitious life problems that can be used in wisdom therapy

Conflicts in the Workplace/Denouncement (P1–P4)	Persons Concerned
P1 Mr. Smith founded an association and invested a lot of work as well as private money. After the association starts to work well, Mr. Smith is ousted and replaced as chairman by a more popular member of the association.	Mr. Smith, the rival, an association member
P2 After being a successful head of department for 25 years, Mr. Smith loses his position due to a work accident and a subsequent stay in hospital. When he comes back he is replaced by a young university graduate.	Mr. Smith, the new boss, the staff manager
P3 Mrs. Miller has been working in a small company side by side with the owner for 28 years with high commitment. When financial problems arise, she is told by letter that she is dismissed. Nobody talks to her.	Mrs. Miller, the owner of the company, a colleague
P4 For 20 years, Mrs. Miller had a leading position in a small bank. When the bank is taken over by another firm, Mrs. Miller's position and salary are reduced to a remarkably lower standard. Her new supervisor is a woman of her daughter's age with less work experience than she has herself.	Mrs. Miller, the new supervisor, the staff manager
Partnership Conflicts (P5–P7)	
P5 In 20 years of marriage, Mrs. Miller took care of the children, the household, and the family's social activities, in order to support her husband's career. Her husband leaves her for his significantly younger assistant whom he believes to be the love of his life.	Mrs. Miller, the husband, the new wife
P6 Mr. Smith is imprisoned because of fraud. After 6 months, his innocence is shown. Meanwhile his wife has left him.	Mr. Smith, the judge, the wife
P7 Mr. Miller tells his wife that he wants to separate because he needs more freedom. A few days later, she hears through a third party that her husband has moved in with one of her female friends with whom he had an affair months earlier.	Mrs. Miller, the husband, the female friend

Table 18. (Continued)

Financial Losses (P8–P10)	Persons Concerned
P8	Mrs. Miller's husband caused a fire which burned down the entire house for which they had been saving money for years. The insurance company does not cover the damage.	Mrs. Miller, the husband, the insurance agent
P9	Mr. Smith was innocently involved in a car accident which caused huge material damage not covered by insurance. The only witnesses to the accident were riding in the other car, so that he was found guilty in court.	Mr. Smith, the driver of the other car, the witness
P10	Ms. Miller was the long-term partner of a chronically ill man, whom she took intensive care of before he passed away. Ms. Miller does not inherit anything while his former wife, who left him for another man, gets all the money.	Ms. Miller, the ill man, the wife
Family Problems, Illness, and Death (P11–P13)	
P11	Ms. Miller, a single mother, had to give up her job to look after her son and his education with great care. After a conflict, the 16-year-old decides to move in with his father who never cared about the family.	Ms. Miller, the son, the father
P12	Mrs. Miller is suffering from rheumatism and in need of help. When this becomes apparent, her husband leaves her for another woman.	Mrs. Miller, her husband, the other woman
P13	Mrs. Miller's 17-year-old son of suffers serious injuries in a car accident. The driver, an 18-year-old friend, was drunk. He is unharmed.	Mrs. Miller, the driver, the son

Training questions for dealing with unsolvable problems

In order to support a structured learning process, the patient can be asked the following questions in relation to such life problems:

1. "Please describe your feelings and thoughts when thinking about this life problem. How does the problem affect you?"

2. Please put yourself into the place of the aggrieved person. How would you feel? What would you think? What would you do?
3. Please put yourself into the place of the originator. How would you feel? What would you think? What would you do?
4. Please put yourself into the place of the third person concerned. What would you think? What would you do?

Question 1 and 2 assess the subjective relevance of the presented life problem. In addition, the patient ought to verbalize and differentiate his/her own negative and positive emotions. This facilitates the perception and acceptance of emotions. Questions 3 and 4 practice the ability to change perspective, and show empathy towards the other persons involved (especially towards the "offender" and their possible motives). Moreover, general knowledge about problem solving is activated. The patient ought to practice looking at problems from the standpoint of different persons with different motives, life situations, and practical constraints, and to reflect on the adequate positive and negative emotions, respectively. This also facilitates value relativism (different values, motives, and life goals of the persons involved can be distinguished, and result in different perspectives and behaviors), as well as contextualism (the temporal and situational embedding of the problem may be reflected). In particular, the behavior of the offender can be discussed and reattributed (specific situational requirements and the enforcement of specific interests can explain specific behavior). Furthermore, the contribution of the aggrieved person to the development of the problem can by brought up. In addition, it may be elaborated that under certain circumstances the patient would have done the same thing as the "offender."

5. Please put yourself into the place of the aggrieved person. What reactions would you consider harmful? Which "solutions" could add insult to injury?

The identified dysfunctional strategies (e.g., self-harm by suicide or alcohol, acts of revenge, long-lasting social and occupational adversities caused by embitterment) may be used to deduce helpful and appropriate options to deal with difficult life problems. Functional strategies that are appropriate for inner processing of injustice, acceptance, and bearing of the insult, as well as active reorientation and development of new perspectives should be reinforced.

6. Which approaches to the problem would you consider reasonable and appropriate for the current situation? Which reactions would be reasonable and appropriate in the long run?

By contrasting short- and long-term consequences, the patient is to become aware that complex life problems always have negative as well as positive consequences, and that it is important to accept these ambivalences.

7. Could you imagine that the presented life problem could have, besides all drawbacks, any positive outcomes for the aggrieved person?

In terms of a long-term perspective, the patient is asked to specifically search for possible positive aspects of the problem (e.g., chance for a new beginning, long-term improvement of life situation due to change, "inner moral growth," and so forth).

8. Please imagine the further development of the aggrieved person. What could their life look like in 5 years from now? How will they reconsider the problem?

Here, an inner spatial and temporaral distance is created from which the patient ought to examine the problem. This opens up the possibility to put the problem into perspective.

9. In the following, five persons are introduced that ought to deal with the problem. What could be typical approaches to difficult life problems for these persons? What would these persons advise?

The persons are: The benevolent grandmother (who got her children through the war, and who has undergone a lot of difficulties); a manager (a rational person who is engaged in practical problem solving); a priest (who is engaged in moral and philosophical questions); a psychologist (who deals with human behavior and problems); an anthropologist (who is engaged in studying the way of life, culture, and habits of people in Africa).

10. Please imagine that, advanced in years, you are writing your biography with all ups and downs of your eventful life. How would you describe and evaluate the current difficult period of life? Is it possible to describe it with more humor and calmness from a distance?

After finishing the first training session, a new life problem that can be similar to the personal problem of the patient is discussed during the next meeting, following the given structure. These questions can be asked explicitly in connection to the patient's personal problem only if the patient shows dedication and cooperation.

3.3 A Case Vignette

The 47-year-old patient is admitted as an inpatient through her health insurance because she had been on sick leave for nine months. She reports suffering from a depressed mood, sleep disorders, fatigue, loss of drive, and multiple somatic symptoms. She had been working in a supermarket and because of her mental state she is no longer able to work and now looking for a sickness pension and early retirement.

Further assessment shows that she really cannot go to work as she reacts with panic when confronted with the idea of visiting her former place of work. She has recently even started to avoid all supermarkets.

When the patient starts to talk about her work, she becomes very upset. She starts to cry and turns to the therapist in an aggressive way because he has asked what would happen if she went to her former workplace. She expresses that the therapist obviously cannot understand her and wants to end the contact.

The therapist starts by telling the patient that he really sees how much she is suffering, that she undoubtedly cannot work or even confront the workplace, and that he suspects that she must have experienced terrible things there. Now the patient starts to complain extensively. She has been threatened with dismissal because a supervisor thinks she has stolen money.

The therapist shows that he is very moved by what he hears und that he is sure that a person like the patient would never take a dime. This is emotionally reiterated by the patient. The therapist also tells the patient that he would be very hurt if somebody thought he was a thief. This is unbelievable, unacceptable, and terrible. And, furthermore, once such a suspicion has been raised, this will never be forgotten. This is what can really drive a person crazy.

The empathic and understanding next question is what has been worst about the whole event. The somewhat surprising answer is that it was the behavior of her immediate boss. She knows that the company sends supervisors to their supermarkets and that these are trying to molest and possibly even fire people. That is how central control is executed nowadays. But her immediate boss has not said a word and by doing so has supported the assumption that she could be a thief. She has worked with him for years, she has always been ready to help out and has helped him in many difficult situations. He should know better and he should have come to her help. Nobody is trustworthy! This report is accompanied by heavy emotional outbursts.

The patient turns out to be a good-natured person, always working, and never cheating. Her view of the world is that you have to work to earn your living and that when you do nothing wrong, nothing wrong will happen to you. Being suspected of theft is the worst thing she can imagine.

The next step is to have a closer look at her feelings. The therapist tells her that he himself is deeply moved by her report. If this happened to him, he would think of revenge. He would deflate the tires of the boss's car or even set fire to the whole supermarket, or at least hope that the supermarket would go bankrupt because of thieves. To this suggestion the patient responds that she would never do anything like this. This is totally against what she thinks one can do. Nevertheless, she starts to grin and a totally new emotional state becomes visible. No, she would not do anything, but to observe the supermarket going bankrupt would really give her a lot of pleasure. The therapist stimulates further emotions of this kind. Would it not be nice to see the boss slip on a banana? The patient discloses that she has had such fantasies herself, but thought that they were unacceptable.

Now the therapist has been very understanding. To be in such a terrible state of mind is horrendous. It is double injustice that they not only spoil her reputation but also rob her of her sleep and good humor. It is not fair that the supervisor and her boss have so much control over her mood and well-being. The patient also thinks that this is doubly injust. She says that she is not only suffering from what has happened but that her present state of mind is also a burden to her. She would love to be able to stop to think constantly about what happened and instead at least once in a while go out and think about something else. But this is impossible. Every supermarket and every advertisement on the TV reminds her of the disaster. And there are many supermarkets and many advertisements. She realizes that she has also become unbearable for her family. She has a good husband. But she wonders how long he will stay at her side as she has become a totally different person. She feels sorry but can do nothing about it.

The question is whether there are situations in which she is distracted for moments. The patient accepts to give it a try. She approaches other patients and actively tries to distract herself at least a little bit.

The question is also how she coped in general or, in particular, with negative life events. How did she react to other problems in her life. What does she know about coping with unbearable life problems? How would she react if she, for example, saw a man leaving his ill wife and looking for a younger one? The patient first reacts to this idea with outrage. This is disdainful. So, how would she comment on such a problem if she imagines that she has met the man of her life who unfortunately is married to a sick woman? She would not break into the marriage although she can understand the temptation.

The personal problem of the patient is moved more and more into the background and instead the question is how people in general handle problems in life, how different people are in their reaction to the same situation, how different their views can be, how much injustice there is and that no-one can escape such experiences. How does one behave honorably in such situations?

The patient learns to discuss such problems from different points of view. She adds examples herself.

This is the time to ask the question which has been deliberately avoided by the therapist until now, why her boss and her colleagues have behaved so unbelievably. Was this because of their bad character? This assumption is rejected by the patient. Instead she suspects that her boss was intimidated and afraid himself. Was he a coward? Possibly, the evidence that she could be a thief was so overwhelming at first sight that he may not have known what to think. After all, the charges had been presented very convincingly and he might have been as perplexed as she was. Did he perhaps want to help, however, did not see this moment as suitable? Was she sure he had said nothing? After all, she herself was very upset at that moment and no longer had a clear view of things. Had she asked him or her colleagues what had really happened? She had until now declined any contact with former colleagues or her boss.

A clarification is needed. What happened? In a micro-analysis, every moment, every reaction, every word, and every emotion is rehearsed. Obviously, her boss was also threatened to be let off as it appeared that he had no control over his staff. The patient looks at the situation from the perspective of her boss. She would possibly also have been silent. The man is even older than she is. If he loses his job, he will never find another. His wife is sick and there are two children.

What can be the next step? The patient thinks that avoidance of supermarkets is most restricting and unnecessary. She decides to actively approach a supermarket run by another company. She also thinks that she should begin to think of her own life. She looks for job opportunities in other supermarkets. She asks herself why she does not think back in the same anger any more. She even has some sympathy for her former boss. Perhaps she should speak to him. She reactivates her old basic values of reliability and honesty, this time towards her boss. She does not want to be unfair to him. She contacts former colleagues. She learns that they were also upset about what had been done to her. When she is dismissed, the patient looks for a new job. She is convinced that she is a good and reliable employee and can introduce herself with self-confidence. The accusation of theft has never been substantiated.

4. References

Abela, J. R. Z., & D'Allessandro, D. U. (2002). Beck's cognitive theory of depression: A test of the diathesis-stress and causal mediation components. *British Journal of Clinical Psychology*, 41, 111–128.

Abelson, R. P. (1963). Computer simulation of "hot cognition." In S. S. Tomkins & S. Mesick (Eds.), *Computer simulations of personality* (pp. 299–302). New York: Wiley.

Achberger, M., Linden, M., Benkert, O. (1999). Psychological distress and psychiatric disorders in primary health care patients in East and West Germany 1 year after the fall of the Berlin wall. *Social Psychiatry & Psychiatric Epidemiology*, 34, 195–201.

Albrecht, S. (2004). *Verbitterung bei Allgemeinarztpatienten auf der Grundlage der „Posttraumatischen Verbitterungsstörung"*. Unpublished diploma thesis.

Alexander, J. (1966). The psychology of bitterness. *International Journal of Psycho-Analysis*, 41, 514–520.

AMDP (1995). *Das AMDP-System. Manual zur Dokumentation psychiatrischer Befunde*. Göttingen: Hogrefe.

American Psychiatric Assosiation (1980). *Diagnostic and statistical manual of mental disorders*. Washington, American Psychiatric Association.

American Psychiatric Assosiation (1994). *Diagnostic and statistical manual of mental disorders* (4th ed.), Washington, American Psychiatric Association.

Andreasen, N. C., Wasek, P. (1980). Adjustment disorders in adolescents. *Archives of General Psychiatry*, 37, 1166–1170.

Antonovsky, A. (1979). *Health, stress, and coping*. San Francisco, CA: Jossey-Bass.

Ardelt, M. (1997). Wisdom and life satisfaction in old age. *The Journals of Gerontology*, 52B, 15–27.

Ardelt, M. (2000a). Antecedents and effects of wisdom in old age: A longitudinal perspective on aging well. *Research on Aging*, 22, 360–94.

Ardelt, M. (2000b). Intellectual versus wisdom-related knowledge: The case for a different kind of learning in the later years of life. *Educational Gerontology: An International Journal of Research and Practice*, 26, 771–89.

Ardelt, M. (2003). Empirical assessment of a three-dimensional wisdom scale. *Research on Ageing*, 25(3), 275–324.

Ardelt, M. (2004). Wisdom as expert knowledge system: A critical review of a contemporary operationalization of an ancient concept. *Human Development*, 47, 257–285.

Ardelt, M. (2005). How wise people cope with crises and obstacles in life. *ReVision: A Journal of Consciousness and Transformation*, 28, 7–19.

Assmann, A. (1994). Wholesome knowledge: Concepts of wisdom in a historical and cross-cultural perspective. In D.L. Fetherman, R.M. Lerner, & M. Perlmutter (Eds.), *Life-span development and behavior* (Vol. 12, pp. 187–224). Hillsdale, N.J.: Lawrence Erlbaum.

Asukai, N., Kato, H., Kawamura, N., Kim, Y., Yamamoto, K., Kishimoto, J., Miyake, Y., & Nishizono-Maher, A. (2002). Reliability and validity of the

Japanese-language version of the Impact of Event Scale-Revised (IES-R-J): Four studies of different traumatic events. *The Journal of Nervous and Mental Disease*, 190, 175–182.

Bacelar, W. T. (1998). *Age differences in adult cognitive complexity: The role of life experiences and personality.* Doctoral Dissertation, Rutgers University, New Brunswick, NJ.

Baltes, P. B. (1993). The aging mind: Potential and limits. *Gerontologist*, 33, 580–594.

Baltes, P. B., & Smith, J. (1990). Weisheit und Weisheitsentwicklung: Prolegomena zu einer psychologischen Weisheitstheorie. *Zeitschrift für Entwicklungspsychologie und Pädagogigische Psychologie*, 22, 95–135.

Baltes, P. B., Smith, J., & Staudinger, U. M. (1992). Wisdom and successful aging. In T. Sonderegger (Ed.), *Nebraska Symposium on Motivation* (Vol. 39, pp. 123–167). Lincoln: University of Nebraska Press.

Baltes, P. B., & Staudinger, U. M. (1993). The search for a psychology of wisdom. *Current Directions in Psychological Science*, 2, 75–80.

Baltes, P. B., Staudinger, U. M., & Lindenberger, U. (1999). Lifespan psychology: Theory and application to intellectual functioning. *Annual Review of Psychology*, 50, 471–507.

Baltes, P. B., & Staudinger, U. M. (2000). Wisdom. A metaheuristic (pragmatic) to orchestrate mind and virtue toward excellence. *American Psychologist*, 55, 122–136.

Baltes, P. B. & Freund, A. M. (2003). The intermarriage of wisdom and selective optimization with compensation: Two meta-heuristics guiding the conduct of life. In C. L. M. Keyes and J. Haidt (Eds.), *Flourishing: Positive psychology and the life well-lived*, 249–73. Washington, American Psychiatric Association.

Baltes, P. B., & Kunzmann, U. (2003). Wisdom. *Psychologist*, 16, 131–133.

Baltes, P. B., & Kunzmann, U. (2004). The two faces of wisdom: Wisdom as a general Theory of knowledge and judgment about excellence in mind and virtue vs. wisdom as everyday realization in people and products. *Human Development*, 47, 290–299.

Bandura, A. (1977). Self-efficacy: Toward a unifying theory of behavioral change. *Psychological Review*, 84, 191–215.

Basoglu, M., Mineka, S., Paker, M., Aker, T., Livanou, M., & Gok, S. (1997). Psychological preparedness for trauma as a protective factor in survivors of torture. *Psychological Medicine*, 27, 1421–1433.

Baumann, K., Kessler, H., & Linden, M. (2005). Die Messung von Emotionen. *Verhaltenstherapie und Verhaltensmedizin*, 26, 169–197.

Baures, M. M. (1996). Letting go bitterness and hate. *Journal of Humanistic Psychology*, 36, 75–90.

Beard, G. M. (1881). *American nervousness, its causes and consequences.* New York: Putnam.

Beck, A. T. (1967). *Depression: Clinical, experimental, and theoretical aspects.* New York: Harper & Row.

Beck, A. T., Rush, A. J., Shaw, B., Emery, G. (1979). *Cognitive therapy of depression*. New York: Guilford.

Beck, A. T. (1983). Cognitive therapy of depression: New perspectives. In: P. J. Clayton & J. E. Barett (Eds.), *Treatment of depression: Old controversies and new approaches*. New York: Raven Press.

Benazzi, F. (2003). Major depressive disorder with anger: a bipolar spectrum disorder? *Psychotherapy and Psychosomatics*, 72, 300–306.

Ben-Zur, H., & Zeidner, M. (1991). Anxiety and bodily symptoms under the threat of missile attacks: The Israeli scene. *Anxiety Research*, 4, 79–95.

Bianachi, E. C. (1994). *Elder wisdom. Crafting your own elderhood*. New York: Crossroad.

Birren, J. E., & Fisher, L. M. (1990). The elements of wisdom: Overview and integration. In R. J. Sternberg (Ed.), *Wisdom: Its nature, origins, and development* (pp. 317–332). New York: Cambridge University Press.

Blake, D. D. & Sonnenberg, R. T. (1998). Outcome research on behavioral and cognitive-behavioral treatments for trauma survivors. In: V. M. Follette, J. I. Ruzek, & F. R. Abueg (Eds.), *Cognitive-behavioral therapies for trauma* (pp.15–47). New York: The Guilford Press.

Blanchard, E. B., Hickling, E. J., Buckley, T. C., Taylor, A. E., Vollmer, A., Loos, W. R.(1996). Psychophysiology of posttraumatic stress disorder related to motor vehicle accidents: replication and extension. *Journal of Consulting and Clinical Psychology*, 64, 742–751.

Böhmig-Krumhaar, S. A. (1998). Leistungspotentiale wert-relativierenden Denkens: Die Rolle einer wissensaktivierenden Gedächtnisstrategie. *Berlin, Max-Planck-Institut für Bildungsforschung Studien und Berichte*, Bd. 65.

Böhmig-Krumhaar, S. A., Staudinger, U. M., & Baltes, P. B. (2002). Mehr Toleranz tut Not: Lässt sich wert-relativierendes Wissen und Urteilen mit Hilfe einer wissensaktivierenden Gedächtnisstrategie verbessern? *Zeitschrift für Entwicklungspsychologie und Pädagogische Psychologie*, 34, 30–43.

Bolby, J. (1969). *Attachment and loss: Vol. 1 Attachment*. New York: Basic Books.

Bronisch, T., & Hecht, H. (1989). Validity of adjustment disorder: comparison with major depression. *Journal of Affective Disorders*, 17, 229–236.

Bronisch, T. (1991). Adjustment reactions: a long-term prospective and retrospective follow-up of former patients in a crisis intervention ward. *Acta Psychiatrica Scandinavica*, 84, 86–93.

Brown, G. W. & Harris, T. O. (1978). *Social origins of depression: A study of psychiatric disorder in women*. New York: Free Press.

Brown, M. A. & Munford, A. (1984). Rehabilitation of Post MI depression and psychological invalidism: A pilot study. *International Journal of Psychological Medicine*, 13, 291–298.

Brown, G. W., Bifulco, A., & Harris, T. O. (1987). Life events, vulnerability and onset of depression. *British Journal of Psychiatry*, 150, 30–42.

Brown, G. W. & Harris, T. O. (1989) (Eds.), *Life Events and Illness*. London: Guilford Press.

Cannon, W. B. (1929). *Bodily changes in pain, hunger, fear and rage.* New York: Appelton and Company.

Casey, P., Dorwick, C., Wilkinson, G. (2001) Adjustment disorders: Fault line in the psychiatric glossary. *British Journal of Psychiatry*, 179, 479–481.

Cattell, R. B. (1966). The scree test for the number of factors. *Multivariate Behavioral Research*, 1, 245–276.

Chen, H., Bierhals, A.J., Prigerson, H. G., Kasl, S. V., Mazure, C. M., Jacobs, S. (1999) Gender differences in the effects of bereavement-related psychological distress in health outcomes. *Psychological Medicine*, 29, 369–380.

Chi, M. T. H., Glaser, R., & Rees, E. (1982). Expertise in problem solving. In R. J. Sternberg (Ed.), *Advances in the psychology of human intelligence* (Vol. 1, pp. 7–76). Hillsdale, NJ: Erlbaum.

Chinen, A. B. (1984). Modal logic: A new paradigm of development and late-life potential. *Human Development*, 27, 42–56.

Clayton, V. (1975). Erickson's theory of human development as it applies to the aged: Wisdom as contradictory cognition. *Human Development*, 18, 119–128.

Clayton, V. (1976). *A multidimensional scaling analysis of the concept of wisdom.* Unpublished doctoral dissertation, University of Southern California, Los Angeles.

Clayton, V. (1982). Wisdom and intelligence: The nature and function of knowledge in the later years. *International Journal of Aging and Development*, 15, 315–323.

Clayton, V., & Birren, J. E. (1980). The development of wisdom across the life span: A reexamination of an ancient topic. In P. B. Baltes & J. O. G. Brim (Eds.), *Life-span development and behavior* (Vol. 3, pp. 103–135). New York: Academic Press.

Cohen, F. (1981). Stress and bodily illness. *Psychiatric Clinics of North America*, 4, 269–286.

Collins, R. l., Taylor, S. E., & Skokan, L. A. (1990). A better world or a shattered vision?: Changes in life perspectives following victimization. *Social Cognition*, 8, 263–85.

Colman, A. M. (2003). *Oxford dictionary of psychology.* New York: Oxford University Press.

Creamer, M., Burgess, P., & Pattison, P. (1992). Reaction to trauma: A cognitive processing model. *Journal of Abnormal Psychology*, 101, 452–459.

Csikszentmihalyi, M., & Rathunde, K. (1990). The psychology of wisdom: An evolutionary interpretation. In R. J. Sternberg (Ed.). *Wisdom: Its nature, origins, and development* (pp. 25–51). New York: Cambridge University Press.

Cwikel, J., & Rosovski, U. (1998). Coping with the stress of immigration among new immigrants to Israel from Commonwealth of Independent States (CIS) who were exposed to Chernobyl: The effect of age. *International Journal of Aging and Human Development*, 46, 305–318.

Davidson, J. R. T., Foa, E. B., Blank, A. S., et al. (1996) Posttraumatic stress disorder. In: T. A. Widiger, A. J. Frances, H. A. Pincus, et al. (Eds.) *DSM-IV sourcebook* (pp. 577–606), vol 2. Washington, DC: American Psychiatric Press.

Dehlinger, E., Ortmann, K. (1992). Zufriedenheit mit dem Gesundheitsstatus in der Bundesrepublik Deutschland und der ehemaligen Deutschen Demokratischen Republik. Ein Vergleich. *Gesundheitswesen*, 54, 88–94.

Derogatis, L. R. (1977). *SCL-90-R, administration, scoring & procedures manual-I for the R(evised) version*. Baltimor: John Hopkins University School of Medicine.

Derogatis, L. R. (1992). *The Symptom Checklist-90-revised*. Minneapolis MN: NCS Assessments.

Despland, J. N., Monod, L., & Ferrero, F. (1995). Clinical relevance of adjustment disorder in DSM-III-R and DSM-IV. *Comprehensive Psychiatry*, 36, 454–460.

Dittmann, K. H. (1991). *Perspektiven der Lebensereignisforschung. Eine kritische Diskussion theoretischer und methodischer Probleme und Lösungsansätze*. Frankfurt am Main: Peter Lang.

Dittmann-Kohli, F., & Baltes, P. B. (1990). Toward a neofunctional conception of adult intellectual development: Wisdom as a prototypical case of intellectual growth. In C. N. Alexander & E. J. Langer (Eds.), *Higher stages of human development. Perspectives on adult growth* (pp. 54–78). New York: Oxford University Press.

Dohrenwend, B. S. & Dohrenwendt B. P. (1974) (Eds.), *Stressful life events: Their nature and effects*. New York: John Wiley & Sons.

Dohrenwend, B. S. & Dohrenwendt B. P. (1974a). A brief introduction to research an stressful life events. In: B. S. Dohrenwend & B. P. Dohrenwend (Eds.), *Life events: Their nature and effects*. New York: John Wiley & Sons.

Donaldson, C. & Lam, D. (2004). Rumination, mood and social problem-solving in major depression. *Psychological Medicine* 34, 1309–1318.

Duden (1985) (Ed.), *Bedeutungswörterbuch*. Mannheim: Dudenverlag.

Ehlers, A., Clark, D. M., Dunmore, E. B., Jaycox, L., Meadows, E., Foa, E. B. (1998). Predicting the response to exposure treatment in PTSD: The role of mental defeat and alienation. *Journal of Traumatic Stress*, 11, 457–471.

Ehlers, A., Maercker, A., Boos, A. (2000). Posttraumatic stress disorder following political imprisonment: The role of mental defeat, alienation, and perceived permanent change. *Journal of Abnormal Psychology*, 109, 45–55.

eLook online dictionary (2005). http://www.elook.org/dictionary/g25.html

Epstein, S. (1973). The self-concept revisited, or a theory of a theory. *American Psychologist*, 28, 404–416.

Epstein, S. (1980). The self-concept: A review and the proposal of an integrated theory of personality. In E. Staub (Ed.), *Personality: Basic issues and current research*. Engelwood Cliffs, NJ: Prentice-Hall.

Epstein, S. (1991). The self-concept, the traumatic neurosis, and the structure of personality. In D. Ozer, J. M. Healy, & A. J. Steward (Eds.), Perspectives on personality (Vol. 3). London: Jessica Kingsley.

Erez, A., & Isen, A. M. (2002). The influence of positive affect on the components of expactancy motivation. *Journal of Applied Psychology*, 87, 1055–1067.

Ericsson, K. A., & Smith, J. (1991) (Eds.), Toward *a general theory of expertise: Prospects and limits*. Cambridge, MA: Cambridge University Press.

Erikson, E. H.(1968). *Identity: Youth and crisis*. New York: Norten.

Erikson, E. H.(1976). *Identität und Lebenszyklus*. Frankfurt: Suhrkamp.

Fabrega, H., Mezzich, & J. E., Mezzich, A. C. (1987). Adjustment disorder as a marginal or transitional illness category in DSM-III. *Archives of General Psychiatry*, 44, 567–572.

Fard, F., Hudgens, R. W., & Welner, A. (1979). Undiagnosed psychiatric illness in adolescents. A prospective and seven year follow-up. *Archives of General Psychiatry*, 35, 279–281.

Filipp, G. (1995). Ein allgemeines Modell für die Analyse kritischer Lebensereignisse. In G. Filipp (Ed.), *Kritische Lebensereignisse* (pp. 3–52). München: Beltz.

Finlay-Jones, R. & Brown, G. W. (1981). Types of stressful life event and the onset of anxiety and depressive disorder. *Psychological Medicine*, 11, 803–815.

Finlay-Jones, R. (1989). Anxiety. In: Brown, G. W. & Harris, T. O. (Eds.), *Life Events and Illness* (pp. 95–112). London: Guilford Press.

Fischer, G., Riedesser, P. (1999) (Eds.), Lehrbuch der Psychotraumatologie. München: Reinhardt.

Fletcher, K. (1988). *Belief systems, exposure to stress, and post-traumatic stress disorder in Vietnam veterans*. Doctoral Dissertation, University of Massachusetts at Amherst.

Follette, V. M. , Ruzek, J. I., Abueg, F. R. (1998). *Cognitive-behavioral therapies for trauma*. New York: Guilford, 1998.

Foster, P., & Oxman, T. (1994). A descriptive study of adjustment disorder diagnoses in general hospital patients. *Irish Journal of Psychological Medicine*, 11, 153–157.

Franke, G. (1995). SCL-90-R: *Die Symptom-Checkliste von Derogatis- Deutsche Version. Manual*. Göttingen: Beltz Test.

Frankl, V. E. (1998). *Logotherapie und Existenzanalyse*. Weinheim: Psychologie Verlags Union.

Franko, D.L., Striegel-Moore, R. H., Brown, K. M., Barton, B. A., McMahon, R. P., Schreiber, G. B., Crawford, P. B., & Daniels, S. R. (2004). Expanding our understanding of the relationship between negative life events and depressive symptoms in black and white adolescent girls. *Psychological Medicine* 34, 1319–1330.

Frazier P. A. (1990). Victim attributions and post-rape trauma. *Journal of Personality and Social Psychology*, 59, 298–304.

Freud, S. (1999). *Jenseits des Lustprinzips*. Frankfurt am Main: Fischer Taschenbuch.

Fullerton, C. S., McCarroll, J. E., Ursano, R. J., Wright, K. M. (1992). Psychological response of rescue workers: firefighters and trauma. *American Journal of Orthopsychiatry*, 62, 371–378.

Gillard, M., & Patton, D. (1999). Disaster stress following a hurricane: The role of religious differences in the Fijian Islands. *The Australasian Journal of Disaster and Trauma Studies*, 2 (Internet publication: http://www.massey.ac.nz/~trauma/ issues/1999-2/gillard.htm).

Goleman, D. (1999). *Emotionale Intelligenz*. München: Deutscher Taschenbuch Verlag.

Greenberg, W. M., Rosenfeld, D. N., & Ortega, E. A. (1995). Adjustment disorder as an admission diagnosis. *American Journal of Psychiatry*, 152, 459–461.

Grimm, J & Grimm, W. (2005) Deutsches Wörterbuch von Jacob und Wilhelm Grimm im Internet. http://germazope.uni-trier.de/Projects/WBB/woerterbuecher/dwb/wbgui?lemid=GV00517

Gottschalk, L. A., Fronczek, J., Abel, L., Buchsbaum, M. S., Fallon, J. H. (2001). The cerebral neurobiology of anxiety, anxiety displacement, and anxiety denial. *Psychotherapy and Psychosomatics*, 70, 17–24.

Häcker, H., & Stapf, K. H. (1998) (Eds.), *Dorsch Psychologisches Wörterbuch*, 13th edition. Bern: Huber.

Hales, R. E., Yudofsky, S. C. & Talbott, J. A. (1999) (Eds.), *Textbook of Psychiatry*, 3rd edition. : Washington: The American Psychiatry Press.

Hall, G. S. (1922). *Senescense: The last half of life*. New York: Appelton.

Hawkes, J. (1857). On the increase of insanity. *Journal of Psychological Medicine and Mental Pathology*, 10, 508–521.

Hawkins, N. G., Davies, R., & Holmes, T. H. (1957). Evidence of psychosocial factors in the development of pulmonary tuberculosis. *American Review of Tuberculosis and Pulmonary Diseases*, 75, 768–780.

Hessel, A., Schumacher, J., Geyer, M. & Brähler, E. (2001) Symptom-Checkliste SCL-90-R: Testtheoretische Überprüfung und Normierung an einer bevölkerungsrepräsentativen Stichprobe. *Diagnostica*, 47, 27–39.

Hillen, T., Schaub, R., Hiestermann, A., Kirschner, W., Robra, B. P. (2000). Self rating of health is associated with stressful life events, social support and residency in East and West Berlin shortly after the fall of the wall. *Journal of Epidemiology and Communal Health*, 54, 575–580.

Holliday, S. G., & Chandler, M. J. (1986). *Wisdom: Explorations in adult competence*. Basel: Karger.

Holmes, T. H. & Masuda, M. (1974). Life Change and Illness Susceptibility. In: B. S. Dohrenwend & B. P. Dohrenwend (Eds.). *Stressful life events: Their nature and effects* (pp. 45–72). New York: John Wiley & Sons.

Holmes, T. H. & Rahe, R. H. (1967). The social readjustment rating scale. *Journal of Psychosomatic Research*, 11, 213–218.

Horowitz, M. J., Wilner, N., & Alvarez, W. (1979) Impact of Event Scale: A measure of subjective stress. *Psychosomatic Medicine*, 41, 209–218.

Isen, A. M. (2001). An influence of positive affect on decision making in complex situations: Theoretical issues with practical implications. *Journal of Consumer Psychology*, 11, 75–86.

Izard, C. E. (2001). Emotional intelligence or adaptive emotions? *Emotion*, 1, 249–257.

Janoff-Bulman, R. (1979). Characterological versus behavioral self-blame: inquiries into depression and rape. *Journal of Personality and Social Psychology*, 37, 1798–1809.

Janoff-Bulman, R. (1985). The aftermath of victimization: Rebuilding shattered assumptions. In Figley (Ed.), *Trauma and its wake*, (Vol. 1). New York: Bruner/Mazel.

Janoff-Bulman, R. (1989). Assumptive world and the stress of traumatic events: Applications of the schema construct. *Social Cognition*, 7, 113–136.

Janoff-Bulman, R. (1990). Understanding people in terms of their assumptive worlds. D. Ozer, J. M. Healy, & A. J. Steward (Eds.), *Perspectives on personality: Self and emotion*. Greenwich, CT: JAI.

Janoff-Bulman, R. (1992). *Shattered assumptions: Towards a new psychology of trauma*. New York: Free Press.

Janoff-Bulman, R. (1998). From terror to appreciation: Confronting chance after extreme misfortune. *Psychological Inquiry*, 9, 99–101.

Janoff-Bulman, R., & Frieze, I. H. (1983). A theoretical perspective for understandingreactions to victimization. *Journal of Social Issues*, 39, 1–17.

Jaspers, K. (1973). *Allgemeine Psychopathologie*. Berlin: Springer-Verlag.

Jones, R., Yates, W. R., Williams, S., Zhou, M., & Hardman, L. (1999). Outcome for adjustment disorder with depressed mood: comparison with other mood disorders. *Journal of Affective Disorders*, 55, 55–61.

Karanci, N. A., Alkan, N., Balta, E., Sucuoglu, H., & Aksit, B. (1999). Gender differences in psychological distress, coping, social support and related variables following the 1995 Dinal (Turkey) earthquake. *North American Journal of Psychology*, 1, 189–204.

Kasl, S.V., Gore, S., & Gore, S. (1975). The experience of losing a job: reported changes in health, symptoms and illness behaviour. *Psychosomatic Medicine*, 37, 106–122.

Kekes, J. (1983). Wisdom. *American Philosophical Quarterly*, 20, 277–286.

Kekes, J. (1995). *Moral wisdom and good lives*. Ithaca, NY: Cornell University Press.

Kelley, G. A. (1955). *The psychology of personal constructs*. New York: Norton.

Kendler, K. S., Karkowski, L.M. & Prescott, C. A. (1999). Causal relationship between stressful life events and the onset of major depression. *American Journal of Psychiatry* 156, 837–848.

Kitschner, K. S., & Brenner, H. G. (1990). Wisdom and reflective judgment: Knowing in the face of uncertainty. In R. J. Sternberg (Ed.), *Wisdom: Its nature, origins, and development* (pp. 212–229). New York: Cambridge University Press.

Kjaer Fuglsang, A., Moergeli, H., Hepp-Beg, S., Schnyder, U. (2001). Who develops acute stress disorder after accident injuries? *Psychotherapy and Psychosomatics*, 71, 214–222.

Kobasa, S C. (1979). Stressful life events, personality, and health: An inquiry into hardiness. *Journal of Personality and Social Psychology*, 37, 1–11.

Kramer, D. A. (1990). Conceptualizing wisdom: The primacy of affect-cognition relations. In R. J. Sternberg (Ed.), *Wisdom: Its nature, origins, and development* (pp. 212–229). New York: Cambridge University Press.

Kramer, D. A. (2000). Wisdom as a classical source of human strength: Conceptualization and empirical inquiry. *Journal of Social and Clinical Psychology*, 19, 83–101.

Krohne, H. W. (2001). Stress and coping theories. In N. J. Smelser & P. B. Baltes (Eds.), *The international encyclopedia of the social and behavioral sciences* (pp. 15163–15170), Vol. 22. Oxford, UK: Elsevier.

Kulka, R., A., Schlenger, W. E. , Fairbank, J. A., Hough, R. L., Jordan, B. K., Marmar, C. R., Weiss, D. S. (1990). *Trauma and the Vietnam War generation. Report of findings from the national Vietnam veterans readjustment study.* New York, Brunner.

Kunzmann, P., Burkard, F.-P., & Wiedemann, F. (1998) *Dtv-Atlas. Philosophie.* München: Deutscher Taschenbuch Verlag.

Kunzmann, U., & Baltes, P. B. (2003). Beyond the traditional scope of intelligence: Wisdom in action. In R. J. Sternberg (Ed.), *Models of intelligence: International perspectives* (pp. 329–343). Washington, DC: American Psychological Association.

Labouvie-Vief, G. (1990). Wisdom as integrated thought: Historical and developmental perspectives. In R. J. Sternberg (Ed.), *Wisdom: Its nature, origins, and development* (pp. 53–83). New York: Cambridge University Press.

Lazarus, R. S. (1966). *Psychological stress and the coping process.* New York: McGraw-Hill.

Leino-Arjas, P., Liira, J., Mutanen, P. Malmivaara, A., Matikainen, E. (1999). Predictors and consequences of unemployment among construction workers: prospective cohort study. *British Medical Journal*, 319, 600–605.

Langenscheid-Longman (1995) (Ed.), *Dictionary of contemporary English.* München: Langenscheid-Longman.

Lehrl, S. (1995). *Mehrfachwahl-Wortschatz-Intelligenztest MWT-B.* Göttingen: Hogrefe.

Lichtenstein, P., Gatz, M., Berg, S. (1998). A twin study of mortality after spouse bereavement. *Psychological Medicine*, 28, 635–643.

Linden M. (2003). The Posttraumatic Embitterment Disorder. *Psychotherapy and Psychosomatics*, 72, 195 – 202.

Linden M. (2004). Posttraumatische Verbitterungsstörung als Folge gesellschaftlichen Umbruchs. In: Bundesärztekammer (Ed.), *Fortschritt und Fortbildung in der Medizin, Band 27* (pp. 77–81). Berlin: Bundesärztekammer.

Linden M., Schippan B., Baumann K., Spielberg R. (2004). Die posttraumatische Verbitterungsstörung (PTED): Abgrenzung einer spezifischen Form der Anpassungsstörungen. *Nervenarzt*, 75, 51–57.

Livanou, M., Basoglu, M., Marks, I., De, S. P., Noshirvani, H., Lovell, K., Thrasher, S. (2002). Beliefs, sense of control and treatment outcome in post traumatic stress disorder. *Psychological Medicine*, 32, 157–165.

Lyster, T. L. (1996). *A nomination approach to the study of wisdom in old age.* Doctoral Dissertation, Concordia University, Montreal, Quebec, Canada.

Madianos, M. G., Papaghelis, M., Ioannovich, J., Dafni, R. (2001). Psychiatric disorders in burn-patients: a follow up study. *Psychotherapy and Psychosomatics*, 70: 30–37.

Maguire, G. P., Lee, E. G., Bevington, D. J., Kuchemann, C. S., Crabtree, R. J., & Cornell, C. E. (1978). Psychiatric problems in the first year after mastectomy. *British Medical Journal*, 319, 600–605.

Magwaza, A. S. (1999). Assumptive world of traumatized South African adults. *Journal of Social Psychology*, 139, 622–630.

Maercker, A. & Schützwohl, M. (1998). Erfassung von psychischen Belastungsfolgen: Die Impact of Event Skala- revidierte Version (IES-R). *Diagnostica*, 44, 130–141.

Maercker, A., Böhmig-Krumhaar, S. A., Staudinger, M. (1998). Existentielle Konfrontation als Zugang zu weisheitsbezogenem Wissen und Urteilen. *Zeitschrift für Entwicklungspsychologie und Pädagogische Psychologie*, 30, 2–12.

Maercker, A, (2003) (Ed.), *Therapie der posttraumatischen Belastungsstörungen.* Berlin: Springer.

Maercker, A. (2003). Erscheinungsbild, Erklärungsansätze und Therapieforschung. In: A. Maerker (Ed.), *Therapie der posttraumatischen Belastungsstörung* (pp. 3–37). Heidelberg: Springer.

Marris, P. (1975). *Loss and change.* Garden City, NY: Anchor/Doubleday.

Marshall, R. D., Spitzer, R., & Liebowitz, M. R. (1999). Review and critique of the new DSM-IV diagnosis of acute stress disorder. *American Journal of Psychiatry*, 156, 1677–1685.

Mason, J. W. (1975). A historical view of the stress field. *Journal of Human Stress*, 1, 22–36.

Matthews, G., Zeidner, M., & Roberts, R. D. (2002). *Emotional intelligence: Science and myth.* Boston: MIT Press.

Matthews, G., Roberts, R. D., & Zeidner, M. (2004). Seven myths about emotional intelligence. *Psychological Inquiry*, 3, 179–196.

Mayer, J. D., & Salovey, P. (1995). Emotional intelligence and the construction and regulation of feelings. *Applied & Preventive Psychology*, 4, 197–208.

Mayer, J. D., & Salovey P. (1997). What is emotional intelligence? In P. Salovey & D. Sluyter (Eds.), *Emotional Development and Emotional Intelligence: Implications for Educators* (pp. 3–31). New York: Basic Books.

Mayer, J. D., Salovey, P., & Caruso, D. R. (2004). Emotional intelligence: Theory, findings, and implications. *Psychological Inquiry*, 3, 197–215.

McFarlane, A. C. (1992). Avoidance and intrusion in posttraumatic stress disorder. *Journal of Nervous & Mental Disease*, 180, 439–445.

McKenzie, N., Marks, I., Liness, S. (2001). Family and past history of mental illness as predisposing factors in post-traumatic stress disorder. *Psychotherapy and Psychosomatics*, 70, 163–165.

Meacham, J. (1990). The loss of wisdom. In R. J. Sternberg (Ed.), *Wisdom: Its nature, origins, and development* (pp. 181–211). New York: Cambridge University Press.

Meyer, A. (1951). The life chart and the obligation of specifying positive data in psychopathological diagnosis. In: E. E. Winters (Ed.), *Medical teaching. The collected papers of Adolph Meyer* (pp. 52–56), vol. III, Baltimore: The Johns Hopkins Press.

Monroe, S. M. & Simons, A. D. (1991). Diathesis-stress theories in the context of life stress research: Implications for the depressive disorders. *Psychological Bulletin*, 110, 406–425.

Muthny, F. A., Gramus, B., Dutton, M., & Stegie, R. (1987). *Tschernobyl- Erlebte Belastung und erste Verarbeitungsversuche*. Weinheim: Studienverlag.

Norris, F. H., Perris, J. L., Ibañez, G. E., & Murphy, A. D. (2001). Sex differences in symptoms of posttraumatic stress: Does culture play a role? *Journal of Traumatic Stress*, 14, 7–28.

Palfai, T. P., & Salovey, P. (1993). The influence of depressed and elated mood on deductive and inductive reasoning. *Imagination, Cognition and Personality*, 13, 57–71.

Parkes, C. M. (1975). What becomes of redundant world models? A contribution to the study of adaptation to change. *British Journal of Medical Psychology*, 48, 131–137.

Pascual-Leone, J. (1990). An essay on wisdom: Toward organismic processes that make it possible. In R. J. Sternberg (Ed.), *Wisdom: Its nature, origins, and development* (pp. 244–278). New York: Cambridge University Press.

Pasquini, M., Picardi, A., Biondi, M., Gaetano, P., Morosini, P. (2004). Relevance of anger and irritability in outpatients with major depressive disorder. *Psychopathology* 37, 155–160.

Pasupathi, M., Staudinger, U. M., & Baltes, P. B. (2001). Seeds of wisdom: Adolescents' knowledge and judgment about difficult life problems. *Developmental Psychology*, 37, 351–361.

Pasupathi, M., Staudinger, U. M., & Baltes, P. B. (1999). The *emergence of wisdom-related knowledge and judgment during adolescence*. Berlin: Max Planck Institute for Human Development.

Patton, G. C., Coffey, C., Posterino, M., Carlin, J. B. & Bowes, G. (2003). Life events and early onset depression: cause or consequence? *Psychological Medicine* 33, 1203–1210.

Paykel, E. S. (1974). Life stress and psychiatric disorder: Applications of the clinical approach. In: B. S. Dohrenwend & B. P. Dohrenwend (Eds.), *Life events: Their nature and effects* (pp. 135–150). New York: John Wiley & Sons.

Paykel, E. S. (1983). Methodological aspects of live events research. *Journal of Psychosomatic research*, 27, 341–352.

Paykel, E. S. (2001a). Stress and affective disorders in humans. *Seminars in Clinical Neuropsychiatry*, 6, 4–11.

Paykel, E. S. (2001b). The evolution of live events research in psychiatry. *Journal of Affective Disorders*, 62, 141–149.

Paykel, E. S. (2003). Life events: effects and genesis. *Psychological Medicine*, 33, 1145–1148.

Petermann, F. (1995). Identifikation und Effektanalyse von kritischen Lebensereignissen. In G. Filipp (Ed.), *Kritische Lebensereignisse* (pp. 53–90), München: Beltz.

Piaget, J. (1972). *The psychology of intelligence*. Totowa, NJ: Littelfield-Adams.

Pirhacova, I. (1997). Perceived social injustice and negative affective states. *Studia Psychologica* 39, 133–136.

Popkin, M. K., Callies, A. L., Colón, E. A., Eduardo, M., & Stiebel, L. (1990). Adjustment disorders in medically ill patients referred for consultation in a university hospital. *Psychosomatics*, 31, 410–414.

Pollock, D. (1992) Structured ambiguity and the definition of psychiatric illness: adjustment disorder among medical inpatients. *Social Sciences and Medicine*, 35, 25–35.

Rahe, R. H., Meyer, M., Smith, M., Kjaer, G., Holmes, T.H., (1964). Social stress and illness onset. *Journal of Psychosomatic Research*, 8, 35–44.

Reck, C. (2001). *Kritische Lebensereignisse und Depression*. Berlin: Lengerich.

Reimer, C. (1995). Tiefenpsychologische Zugänge zu depressiv Kranken. *Psychotherapeut*, 40, 367–372.

Reinecker, H. (2003). Forschung in der Klinischen Psychologie. In H. Reinecker (Ed.), *Lehrbuch der klinischen Psychologie und Psychotherapie. Modelle psychischer Störungen* (pp.23–38). Göttingen: Hogrefe.

Rini, C., Manne, S., DuHamel, K. N., Austin, J., Ostroff, J., Boulad, F., Parsons, S. K., Marini, R., Williams, S., Mee, L., Sexon, S., & Redd, W. H. (2004). Changes in mother's basic beliefs following a child's bone marrow transplantation: The role of prior trauma and negative life events. *Journal of Traumatic Stress*, 17, 325–333.

Ritter, K. (2003).*Globale und differentielle Lebenszufriedenheit: Eine Untersuchung mit dem Differentiellen Lebenszufriedenheitsfragebogen.* Unpublished diploma thesis.

Roberts, J. E., Gilboa, E. & Gotlib, I. H. (1998). Ruminative response style and vulnerability to episodes of dysphoria: gender, neuroticism and episode duration. *Cognitive Therapy and research*, 22, 401–423.

Robinson, D. N. (1989). *Aristotle's psychology*. New York: Columbia University Press.

Robinson, D. N. (1990). Wisdom through the ages. In R. J. Sternberg (Ed.), *Wisdom: Its nature, origins, and development* (pp. 13–24). New York: Cambridge University Press.

Rush, A. J., & Weissenburger, J. E. (1995). Melancholic symptom features and DSM-IV. *American Journal of Psychiatry*, 152, 1242–1243.

Salovey, P., & Mayer J. D. (1990). Emotional intelligence. *Imagination, Cognition, and Personality*, 9, 185–211.

Satzger, W., Fessmann, H., Engel, R. R. (2002). Liefern HAWIE-R, WST und MWT-B vergleichbare IQ-Werte? *Zeitschrift für Differentielle und Diagnostische Psychologie*, 23, 159–170.

Schaad, R. (2002). *Berner Verbitterungs-Bogen (Version 2)*. Lizentiatsarbeit, Institut für Psychologie der Universität Bern.

Scheier, M. F., & Carver, C. S. (1992). Effects of optimism on psychological and physical well-being: Theoretical overview and empirical update. *Cognitive Therapy & Research*, Vol 16, 201–228.

Schippan B., Baumann K., & Linden, M. (2004). Weisheitstherapie – kognitive Therapie der posttraumatischen Verbitterungsstörung. *Verhaltenstherapie*, 14, 284–293.

Schmitz, N., Hartkamp, N., Kiuse, J., Franke, G. H, Reister, G., & Tress, W. (2000). The Symptom Check-List-90-R (SCL-90-R): A German validation study. *Quality of Life Research*, 9, 185–193.

Schnyder, U., Buchi, S., Sensky, T., & Klaghofer, R. (2000). Antonovsky´s sense of coherence: trait or state? *Psychotherapy and Psychosomatics*, 69, 296–302.

Schützwohl, M., & Maercker, A. (2000). Ärgererleben und Ärgerausdrucksverhalten nach Traumatisierung. Ausmaß und Beziehung zu posttraumatischen Belastungsreaktionen nach politischer Inhaftierung in der DDR. *Zeitschrift für klinische Psychologie und Psychotherapie*, 29, 187–194.

Schwartzberg, S. S., & Janoff-Bulman, R. (1991). Grief and the search for meaning: Exploring the assumptive worlds of bereaved college students. *Journal of Social and Clinical Psychology*, 10, 270–288.

Schwarzer, R., & Leppin, A. (1991). Social support and health: A theoretical and empirical overview. *Journal of Social and Personal Relationships*, 8, 99–127.

Schwarzer R, & Jerusalem, M. (1994) (Eds.), *Gesellschaftlicher Umbruch als kritisches Lebensereignis. Psychosoziale Krisenbewältigung von Übersiedlern und Ostdeutschen*. Weinheim: Juventa Verlag.

Schwarzer, R., & Schulz, U. (2002). The role of stressful life events. In A. M. Nezu, C. M. Nezu, & P. A. Geller (Eds.), *Comprehensive handbook of psychology*, Vol. 9: Health psychology. New York: Wiley.

Selye, H. (1956). *The stress of life*. New York: McGraw-Hill.

Shapiro, F. (1989). Efficacy of eye movement desensitization procedure in the treatment of traumatic memories. *Journal of Traumatic Stress*, 2, 199–223.

Shaver, K. G., & Drown, D. (1986). On causality, responsibility, and self-blame: a theoretical note. *Journal of Personality and Social Psychology*, 50, 697–702.

Sheehan, D. V., Lecrubier, Y., Sheehan, K. H., Amorim, P., Janavas, J., Weiller, E., Hergueta, T., Baker, R. & Dunbar, G. C. (1998). The Mini-International Neuropsychiatric Interview (M.I.N.I.): The development and validation of a structured diagnostic interview for DSM-IV and ICD-10. *Journal of Clinical Psychiatry*, 59, 22–33.

Shelley, M. (1994). *Frankenstein*. London: Penguin.

Shoda, Y., Mischel, W. & Peake, Ph. K. (1990): Predicting adolescent cognitive and self-regulatory competencies from preschool delay of gratification. *Developmental Psychology*, 26, 978–986.

Smith, J., & Baltes, P. B. (1990). Wisdom-related knowledge: Age/cohort differences in response to life-planning problems. *Developmental Psychology*, 26, 494–505.

Smith, E. E., Bem, D. J., & Nolen-Hoeksema, S. (2001) *Fundamentals of Psychology*. Orlando: Harcourt College Publishers.

Snyder, S., Strain, J. J., & Wolf, D. (1990). Differentiating major depression from adjustment disorder with depressed mood in the medical setting. *General Hospital Psychiatry*, 12, 159–165.

Stampfl, T. G. & Lewis, D. J. (1967). Essentials of implosive therapy: A learning theory based on psychodynamic behavioral therapy. *Journal of Abnormal Psychology*, 72, 496–503.

Strain. J. J., Newcorn, J., Fulop, G., & Sokolyanskaya, M. (1999). Adjustment disorder. In R. E. Hales, S. C. Yudofsky, J. A. Talbott (Eds.), *Textbook of psychiatry* (pp. 759–771), third edition. Washington, DC: American Psychiatric Press.

Staudinger, U. M., Smith, J., & Baltes, P. B. (1992). Wisdom-related knowledge in life review task: Age differences and the role of professional specialization. *Psychology and Aging*, 7, 271–281.

Staudinger, U. M. & Baltes, P. B. (1996a). Weisheit als Gegenstand psychologischer Forschung. *Psychologische Rundschau*, 47, 1–21.

Staudinger, U. M. & Baltes, P. B. (1996b). Interactive minds: A facilitative setting for wisdom-related performance? *Journal of Personality and Social Psychology*, 71, 746–762.

Staudinger, U. M., Lopez, D., & Baltes, P. B (1997). The psychometric location of wisdom-related performance: Intelligence, personality, and more? *Personal and Social Psychological Bulletin*, 23, 1200–1214.

Staudinger, U. M. (1999). Older and wiser? Integrating Results on the relationship between age and wisdom-related performance. *International Journal of Behavioral Development*, 23, 641–664.

Staudinger, U. M., Freund, A. M., Linden, M., & Maas, I. (1999). Self, personality, and life regulation: Facets of psychological resilience in old age. In: Baltes, P. B., Mayer, K. U. (Eds.), *The Berlin Aging Study. Aging from 70 to 100* (pp. 302–328). Cambridge: Cambridge University Press.

Sternberg, R. J. (1982) (Ed.), *Advances in the psychology of human intelligence*. Hillsdale, NJ: Erlbaum.

Sternberg, R. J. (1985). Implicit theories of intelligence, creativity, and wisdom. *Journal of Personality and Social Psychology*, 49, 607–627.

Sternberg, R. J. (1998). A balance theory of wisdom. *Review of General Psychology*, 2, 347–365.

Sternberg, R. J. (1990) (Ed.), *Wisdom: Its nature, origins, and development*. Cambridge: Cambridge University Press.

Stickgold, R. (2002). EMDR: a putative neurobiological mechanism of action. *Journal of Clinical Psychology*, 58, 61–75.

Susemihl, F. (1912) (Ed.), *Aristotelis Ethica Nicomachea*. Leipzig: Apelt.

Tausch, R. (1992). Vergeben, ein bedeutsamer seelischer Vorgang. *Zeitschrift für Sozialpsychologische und Gruppendynamik in Wirtschaft und Gesellschaft*, 17, 3–29.

Taylor, S. E. (1983). Adjustment to threatening events: A theory of cognitive adaptation. *American Psychologist*, 38, 1161–1173.

Timko, C., Janoff-Bulman, R. (1985). Attributions, vulnerability, and psychological adjustment: the case of breast cancer. *Health Psychology*, 4, 521–544.

Toukmanian, S. G., Jadaa, D., & Lawless, D. (2000). A cross-cultural study of depression in the aftermath of a natural disaster. *Anxiety, Stress, and Coping*, 13, 289–307.

Ullrich de Muynck, R. & Ullrich, R. (1976). *Das Assertiveness Training Programm (3 Teile)*. München: Pfeiffer.

Valliant, G. E. (1993). *The wisdom of the ego*. Cambridge, MA: Harvard University Press.

Van der Kolk, B. A., Herron, N., Hostetler, A. (1994). The history of trauma in psychiatry. *Psychiatric Clinics of North America*, 17, 583–600.

Van der Kolk, B. A., McFarlane, A. C., Weisaeth, L. (1996) (Eds.). *Traumatic stress*. New York: Guilford.

Webster, J. D. (1993) Construction and Validation of the Reminiscence Functions Scale. *Journal of Gerontology*, 48, 256–262.

Weiss, D. S., & Marmar, C. R. (1997). The Impact of Event Scale-Revised. In J. P. Wilson & T. M. Keane (Ed), *Assessing psychological trauma and PTSD* (pp. 399–411). New York: Guilford Pree.

Winkler, G. (2002). *Sozialreport*. Berlin: Sozialwissenschaftliches Forschungszentrum Berlin Brandenburg.

Wirtz, M. (2004). Über das Problem fehlender Werte: Wie der Einfluss fehlender Informationen auf Analyseergebnisse entdeckt und reduziert werden kann. *Rehabilitation* 43, 109–115.

Wittchen, H. U., Müller, N., Pfister, H., Winter, S., Schmidtkunz, B. (1999): Affektive, Somatisierungs- und Angsterkrankungen in Deutschland. *Gesundheitswesen*, 61, 216–222.

Wolpe, J. (1958). *Psychotherapy of reciprocal inhibition*. Stanford: University Press.

World Health Organization (1992) (Ed.). *International statistical classification of diseases and related health problems*. 10th Revision. Geneva: WHO.

Zemperl, J. & Frese, M. (1997). Arbeitslose: Selbstverwaltung überwindet die Lethargie. *Psychologie Heute* 24, 36–41.

Zajonc, R. B. (1980). Feeling and thinking: Preferences need no inferences. *American Psychologist*, 35, 151–175.

Znoj, H. (2002). *Der Berner Verbitterungsfragebogen*. Unpuplished.

5. Appendix

PTED Self-Rating Scale

Please read the following statements and indicate to what degree they apply to you. Please do not miss a line.

I agree with this statement

During the last years there was a severe and negative life event	not true at all	hardly true	partially true	very much true	extremely true
1. that hurt my feelings and caused considerable embitterment	0	1	2	3	4
2. that led to a noticeable and persistent negative change in my mental well-being	0	1	2	3	4
3. that I see as very unjust and unfair	0	1	2	3	4
4. about which I have to think over and over again	0	1	2	3	4
5. that causes me to be extremely upset when I am reminded of it	0	1	2	3	4
6. that triggers me to harbor thoughts of revenge	0	1	2	3	4
7. for which I blame and am angry with myself	0	1	2	3	4
8. that led to the feeling that it is pointless to strive or to make an effort	0	1	2	3	4
9. that makes me frequently feel sullen and unhappy	0	1	2	3	4
10. that impaired my overall physical well-being	0	1	2	3	4
11. that causes me to avoid certain places or persons so as not to be reminded of them	0	1	2	3	4
12. that makes me feel helpless and disempowered	0	1	2	3	4
13. that triggers feelings of satisfaction when I think of the responsible party having to experience a similar situation	0	1	2	3	4
14. that led to a considerable decrease in my strength and drive	0	1	2	3	4
15. that caused me to be more easily irritated than before	0	1	2	3	4
16. that has resulted in me having to distract myself in order to experience a normal mood	0	1	2	3	4
17. that made me unable to pursue occupational and/or family activities as before	0	1	2	3	4
18. that caused me to draw back from friends and social activities	0	1	2	3	4
19. which frequently evokes painful memories	0	1	2	3	4

From: Linden, Rotter, Baumann, Lieberei, *Posttraumatic Embitterment Disorder*   Hogrefe & Huber Publishers 2007

Diagnostic Core Interview and Algorithm for PTED

A. Core Criteria		
1. During the last years, was there a severe event/experi-ence that led to a noticeable and persistent negative change in your mental well-being?	→ NO	YES
2. Did you experience the critical life event as unjust or unfair?	→ NO	YES
3. Do you feel embitterment, rage, and helplessness when reminded of the event?	→ NO	YES
4. Did you suffer from any (substantial/relevant/notice-able) psychological or mental problems (depression, anxieties or the like) prior to the event?	NO	→ YES
EVALUATION BY THE EXAMINER:		
EMOTIONAL EMBITTERMENT (MARKED BY EMBITTERMENT, RAGE, AND HELPLESSNESS)?	→ NO	YES
CAN ANY PREMORBID MENTAL DISORDER EXPLAIN THE PRESENT PSYCHOPATHOLOGY?	NO	→ YES
5. For how long have you already suffered from psychological impair-ment caused by the event? (Specify in months.)		
_____ Months	→ Less than 6 months	

From: Linden, Rotter, Baumann, Lieberei, *Posttraumatic Embitterment Disorder*　　© Hogrefe & Huber Publishers 2007

B. Additional Symptoms

1. During the last months, did you repeatedly have intrusive and incriminating thoughts about the event?   NO   YES

2. Does it still extremely upset you when you are reminded of the event?   NO   YES

3. Does the critical event or its originator make you feel helpless and disempowered?   NO   YES

4. Is your prevailing mood since the critical event frequently down?   NO   YES

5. If you are distracted, are you able to experience a normal mood?   NO   YES

ARE FOUR QUESTIONS IN SECTION B
ANSWERED WITH YES?   →
NO   YES

POSTTRAUMATIC EMBITTERMENT DISORDER

NO   YES

ONLY INDICATE YES IF NO PSYCHOLOGICAL DISORDER WAS PRESENT DURING THE YEAR BEFORE THE EVENT.

Note. The Answers marked with an arrow indicate that one of the essential criteria for the diagnosis of PTED is not met. Thus, the clinician is asked to directly indicate "NO" in the diagnostic box at the bottom of the interview.

From: Linden, Rotter, Baumann, Lieberei, *Posttraumatic Embitterment Disorder*   © Hogrefe & Huber Publishers 2007

Clinical Semi–Standardized Diagnostic Interview for PTED

1. During the last years, was there a severe event/experience that *hurt* your feelings *very much* and caused *considerable embitterment*? (Is there more than one event/ experience that comes to your mind?) If yes, please describe them and indicate the year in which they happened.

               ( ) yes   →
               ( ) yes   ( ) no

If Yes: 1.

              2.

              3.

     Other Events:

2. Please indicate the event/experience from the list in question 1 that has been the most important for you in causing your present state of mind and mental well-being.

Critical life event:

3. Did the event lead to a *clear* and *persistent* negative change in your mental well-being?

                                         →
               ( ) yes   ( ) no

4. Did you experience the critical life event as unjust? Do you have the feeling that destiny or the responsible person has treated you unfairly?

               ( ) yes   ( ) no

5. During the last months, did you repeatedly have *intrusive* and incriminating thoughts about the event?

               ( ) yes   ( ) no

6. Does it still extremely upset you, when you are reminded of the event?

               ( ) yes   ( ) no

From: Linden, Rotter, Baumann, Lieberei, *Posttraumatic Embitterment Disorder*   Hogrefe & Huber Publishers 2007

7. Prior to the event, did you suffer from any (substantial/relevant/noticeable) psychological or mental problems (depression, anxieties or the like)?

( ) yes   ( ) no

If so, what kind of problems did you have?

8. Who would you say is responsible for the critical life event (e.g., your boss, a relative, fate, or the like)?

1.

2.

3.

9. Does the critical event or its originator make you fell *helpless* and disempowered?

( ) yes   ( ) no

10. Would it be *satisfying* if the responsible party had to *experience a similar situation*?

( ) yes   ( ) no

11. Would it be *satisfying* if the responsible party were *called to account*?

( ) yes   ( ) no

12. If the critical event is brought up or you have to think about it, does that *trigger the following feelings*?

a) Despair: ( ) yes   ( ) no

b) Hopelessness: ( ) yes   ( ) no

c) Rage: ( ) yes   ( ) no

From: Linden, Rotter, Baumann, Lieberei, *Posttraumatic Embitterment Disorder*   Hogrefe & Huber Publishers 2007

d) Anxiety: ( ) yes   ( ) no

e) Aggression: ( ) yes   ( ) no

f) Embitterment: ( ) yes   ( ) no

g) Sadness: ( ) yes   ( ) no

h) Helplessness: ( ) yes   ( ) no

i) Concern: ( ) yes   ( ) no

j) Anger: ( ) yes   ( ) no

k) Offendedness: ( ) yes   ( ) no

l) Grudge: ( ) yes   ( ) no

m) Humiliation: ( ) yes   ( ) no

n) Shame: ( ) yes   ( ) no

13. Following the critical event, did you *blame yourself*, or are you angry with yourself?

                               ( ) yes   ( ) no

14. Is your prevailing *mood* since the critical event frequently *down*?

                               ( ) yes   ( ) no

15. Is your prevailing mood since the critical event frequently *irritable*?

                               ( ) yes   ( ) no

16. If you are *distracted*, are you able to experience a *normal mood*?

                               ( ) yes   ( ) no

From: Linden, Rotter, Baumann, Lieberei, *Posttraumatic Embitterment Disorder*   Hogrefe & Huber Publishers 2007

17. Since the critical event, have you suffered increasingly from the following affective disturbances?

a) Loss of interest, or loss of enjoyment in engaging in delightful activities:

( ) yes   ( ) no

b) Loss of ability to react emotionally to joyful events:

( ) yes   ( ) no

c) Early awakening:

( ) yes   ( ) no

d) Low mood, especially in the morning:

( ) yes   ( ) no

e) Inhibition of drive:

( ) yes   ( ) no

f) Agitation:

( ) yes   ( ) no

g) Loss of appetite:

( ) yes   ( ) no

h) Loss of weight:

( ) yes   ( ) no

i) Decrease in sexual interest:

( ) yes   ( ) no

18. Since the event, do you often have the feeling that it is *pointless to strive* or to make an effort?

( ) yes   ( ) no

From: Linden, Rotter, Baumann, Lieberei, *Posttraumatic Embitterment Disorder*   Hogrefe & Huber Publishers 2007

19. Do you *avoid places or persons* that could remind you of the critical event?

            ( ) yes   ( ) no

20. Does your emotional state of mind *block family activities*?

            ( ) yes   ( ) no

21. Does your emotional state of mind *block occupational activities*?

            ( ) yes   ( ) no

22. Does your emotional state of mind *block social or leisure time activities*?

            ( ) yes   ( ) no

23. For how long have you already suffered from psychological impairment caused by the event? (Specify in months.)

                           _____ Months

Note. The Answers marked with an arrow indicate that one of the essential criteria for the diagnosis of PTED is not met. If these prerequisites are not met, the patient is estimated as not suffering from PTED. The interview does not need to be continued.

From: Linden, Rotter, Baumann, Lieberei, *Posttraumatic Embitterment Disorder*   Hogrefe & Huber Publishers 2007

Wisdom Rating Scale

Introduction

Life is often unfair. There are many different ways in which people react to such life events. In the following, you will find a fictitious life problem. We would like to know what you think about this situation. Could please give us your comments? Please specify how you would try to cope with this problem, if you were the person concerned. Please take time to think about it.

> Mr. Smith is imprisoned because of fraud. After 6 months, his innocence is shown. Meanwhile his wife has left him.

To what degree does this life problem affect you?

0	1	2	3	4
not at all	hardly	partially	noticeable	strongly

What might one take into consideration and do in such a situation? Please reflect, speak out, and discuss whatever comes to your mind.

The interviewer listens to the person, to what they are saying, to the emotional reaction, to the content and structure of reasoning and makes the following "Ratings of Wisdom-Related Performance":

1. Change of Perspective
To what extent does the person show that the different perspectives of the concerned persons are recognized?

0	1	2	3	4
not at all		partially		very much

2. Empathy
To what extent does the person show that the emotions of the different concerned persons are empathically recognized?

0	1	2	3	4
not at all		partially		very much

From: Linden, Rotter, Baumann, Lieberei, *Posttraumatic Embitterment Disorder*   © Hogrefe & Huber Publishers 2007

3. Acceptance of Emotions
To what extent does the person show that one's own emotions are recognized and accepted?

0	1	2	3	4
not at all		partially		very much

4. Serenity
To what extent does the person show that different perspectives and arguments are reported in an emotionally balanced way?

0	1	2	3	4
not at all		partially		very much

5. Factual Knowledge and Procedural Knowledge
To what extent does the person show general and specific (e.g., life events, variations, institutions) knowledge about life matters and consider strategies of decision making (e.g., cost-benefit analysis), and problem solving?

0	1	2	3	4
not at all		partially		very much

6. Contextualism
To what extent does the person consider the past, current, and possible future contexts of life and the many circumstances in which a life is embedded?

0	1	2	3	4
not at all		partially		very much

7. Value Relativism
To what extent does the person consider variations in values and life priorities and the importance of viewing each person within their own framework of values and life goals, despite a small set of universal values?

0	1	2	3	4
not at all		partially		very much

From: Linden, Rotter, Baumann, Lieberei, *Posttraumatic Embitterment Disorder*   © Hogrefe & Huber Publishers 2007

8. Uncertainty Acceptance

To what extent does the person consider the inherent uncertainty of life (in terms of interpreting the past, predicting the future, managing the present) and effective strategies for dealing with uncertainty?

0	1	2	3	4
not at all		partially		very much

9. Long-Term Perspective

To what extent does the person consider that each behavior can have positive and negative, as well as short- and long-term consequences, which can also contradict each other?

0	1	2	3	4
not at all		partially		very much

Wisdom Training Outline

1. Fictitious Problems and Negative Life Events

This is a list of negative life events. Each event involves three persons. All events are unjust and irreversible for one of the parties involved. They refer to work, family, or other areas of life. For training purposes, it is recommended to select a problem which is different from the problems of the patient. If the patient has suffered from humiliation at work, a family problem can be selected.

Conflicts in the Workplace	Persons Involved
W1 After being a successful head of department for 25 years, Mr. Smith looses his position due to a work accident and a subsequent stay in hospital. When he comes back, he is replaced by a young university graduate.	Mr. Smith, the new boss, the staff manager
W2 Mrs. Miller has been working in a small company side by side with the owner for 28 years with high commitment. When financial problems arise, she is told by letter that she is dismissed and nobody talks to her, while a younger colleague stays in her job.	Mrs. Miller, the owner, a colleague
W3 For 20 years, Mrs. Miller had a leading position in a small bank. When the bank is taken over by another firm, Mrs. Miller's position and salary are reduced to a remarkably lower standard. Her new supervisor is a woman of her daughter's age with less work experience than she has herself.	Mrs. Miller, the new supervisor, the staff manager

Partnership and Family	
P1 In 20 years of marriage, Mrs. Miller took care of the children, the household, and the family's social activities, in order to support her husband's career. Her husband leaves her for his significantly younger assistant whom he believes to be the love of his life.	Mrs. Miller, the husband, the new wife
P2 Mrs. Miller is suffering from breast cancer and is in the need of help. Her husband leaves her for another woman	Mrs. Miller the husband the other woman
P3 Mr. Miller tells his wife that he wants to separate because he needs more freedom. A few days later, she hears through a third party that her husband has moved in with one of her female friends with whom he had an affair months earlier.	Mrs. Miller, the husband, the other woman

From: Linden, Rotter, Baumann, Lieberei, *Posttraumatic Embitterment Disorder*   © Hogrefe & Huber Publishers 2007

P4	Ms. Miller, a single mother, had to give up her job to look after her son and his education with great care. After a conflict, the 16-year-old decides to move in with his father who never cared about the family.	Ms. Miller, the son, the father
P5	Mrs. Miller's 17-year-old son suffers serious injuries in a car accident. The driver, an 18-year-old friend, was drunk. He is unharmed.	Mrs. Miller, the driver, the son

Financial Losses

F1	Mrs. Miller's husband caused a fire which burned down the entire house for which they had been saving money for years. The insurance company does not cover the damage.	Mrs. Miller, the husband, the insurance agent
F2	Mr. Smith was innocently involved in a car accident which caused huge material damage not covered by insurance. The only witnesses to the accident were riding in the other car, so that he was found guilty in court.	Mr. Smith, the driver of the other car, the witness
F3	Mrs. Miller would have hit the jackpot in the lottery, however, she did not get anyhing, as her husband had not handed in the lottery coupon because he spent the money in the pub with his friend.	Mrs. Miller her husband the friend
F4	Mrs. Miller was the long-term partner of a chronically ill man, whom she took intensive care of before he passed away. Mrs. Miller does not inherit anything while his former wife, who left him for another man, gets all the money.	Mrs. Miller, the ill man, the wife

Social Life and Leisure

S1	Mr. Smith founded an association and invested a lot of work as well as private money. After the association starts to work well, Mr. Smith is ousted and replaced as chairman by a more popular member of the association.	Mr. Smith, the rival, an association member
S2	Mr. Miller reads in the newspaper that he is involved in criminal activities, although he is fully innocent. In his club, people turn against him.	Mr. Miller, the journalist, a club member

2. Introduction to the Patient

In the next step, we would like to ask you to look at life problems from different perspectives and through the eyes of another person. Scientific research has confirmed that such a change of perspective is an important way of finding solutions for problems which seem to be unsolvable at first glance. To discover ways out of the difficult situation is another form of intelligence which can be learned.

In the following, different fictitious life problems will be presented to you, and we would like you to consider this situation from the perspective of various people. Furthermore, we would like you to consider beneficial and less beneficial ways of coping with the respective problem in each situation.

Please read the following problem, than answer the subsequent questions. Please take your time to think about the problem.

3. Questions to the Patient

In order to support a structured learning process, the patient can be asked the following questions in relation to such life problems:
1. "Please describe your feelings and thoughts when thinking about this life problem. How does the problem affect you?"
2. Please put yourself into the place of the aggrieved person. How would you feel? What would you think? What would you do?
3. Please put yourself into the place of the originator. How would you feel? What would you think? What would you do?
4. Please put yourself into the place of the third person. What would you think? What would you do?
5. Please put yourself into the place of the aggrieved person. What reactions would you consider as harmful? Which "solutions" could add insult to injury? Which "solutions" would lead to everything turning out even worse?
6. Which approaches to solving the problem would you consider reasonable and appropriate for the current situation?
7. Which reactions would be reasonable and appropriate in the long run?
8. Could you imagine that the presented life problem could have, besides all drawbacks, any positive outcomes for the aggrieved person?
9. Please imagine the further development of the aggrieved person. What could their life look like in 5 years from now? How will they reconsider the problem?
10. Please imagine that, advanced in years, you are writing your biography with all ups and downs of your eventful life. How would you describe and evaluate the current difficult period of life? Is it possible to describe it with more humor and calmness from a distance?

From: Linden, Rotter, Baumann, Lieberei, *Posttraumatic Embitterment Disorder*   © Hogrefe & Huber Publishers 2007

4. Expert Perspectives

In the following, different persons are introduced who can be called experts in the management of life problems. What could be typical approaches to difficult life problems for these persons?

Grandmother
The benevolent grandmother who got her children through the war and who has undergone a lot of difficulties.

Manager
A rational person who is engaged in practical problem solving.

Priest
A person who is engaged in moral and philosophical questions.

Psychologist
A person who deals with human behavior and problems.

Anthropologist
A person who is engaged in studying the way of life, culture, and habits of people in Africa.

4.1.
What could be typical approaches of these persons to solving difficult life problems?

4.2.
What advice would these persons give?

4.3.
What would they do if they had to deal with the life problem of Mrs. Miller or Mr. Smith?

4.4.
Can you come up with "solutions" in connection to the presented life problem, which the experts (grandmother, manager, priest, psychologist, and anthropologist) would consider unreasonable, harmful, or wrong?

From: Linden, Rotter, Baumann, Lieberei, *Posttraumatic Embitterment Disorder*   © Hogrefe & Huber Publishers 2007

5. Personal Problem and Negative Life Event

The personal problem should only be addressed after the patient has shown that they feel that the problem is not only what has happened to them but also how they respond to the problem.

5.1.
Information to the patient:

Please write down in one or two keywords your difficulties (e.g., problems or events) that contribute to or caused your present negative state of mind.

_____

_____

_____

5.2.
To what degree does this life problem affect you?

0	1	2	3	4
not at all	hardly	partially	noticeable	strongly

5.3.
Who are the persons involved in the problem? Who is the originator of the problem? Who is responsible?

5.4.
Who is suffering besides you?

5.5.
Please describe how you have so far tried to cope with the above mentioned difficulties, which have contributed to your present hospitalization. Please take your time to think about it and reflect out loud.

5.6.
Please put yourself into the place of the originator. How would you feel? What would you think? What would you do?

5.7.
Please put yourself into the place of one of the persons who are suffering from the event. What do they think? How do they react?

From: Linden, Rotter, Baumann, Lieberei, *Posttraumatic Embitterment Disorder*   © Hogrefe & Huber Publishers 2007

5.8.
What reactions would you consider as harmful? Which "solutions" could add insult to injury? Which "solutions" would lead to everything turning out even worse?

5.9.
What approaches to solving the problem would you consider reasonable and appropriate for the current situation?

5.10.
Which reactions would be reasonable and appropriate in the long run?

5.11.
Could you imagine that the presented life problem could have, besides all drawbacks, any positive outcomes for you?

5.12.
Please look into the future. What could your life look like in 5 years from now? How will you reconsider the problem?

5.13.
Please imagine that, advanced in years, you are writing your biography with all ups and downs of your eventful life. How would you describe and evaluate the current difficult period of life? Is it possible to describe it with more humor and calmness from a distance?

5.14.
Imagine the five expert persons (grandmother, manager, priest, psychologist, and anthropologist) had exactly the same problems as you do. How would they (respectively) cope with those problems? Please take your time to think about it.

5.15.
Please imagine someone (e.g., parent, friend, acquaintance, relative, politician, or movie hero) who is a model for you when it comes to dealing with difficult life problems or who you would consider a "wise" person. Who is this person?

What are the differences between their strategies and yours? Please take your time to think about it.

5.16.
Do you know someone of whom you are pretty certain that they would find an unreasonable, harmful, or wrong "solution" to any difficult life problem?

What are the differences between their strategies and yours? Please take your time to think about it.

From: Linden, Rotter, Baumann, Lieberei, *Posttraumatic Embitterment Disorder*   © Hogrefe & Huber Publishers 2007

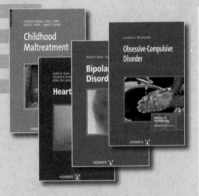
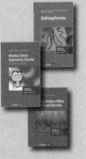
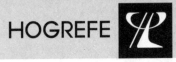

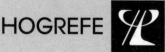

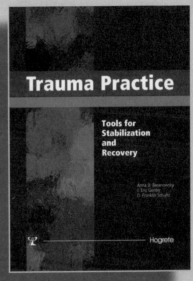
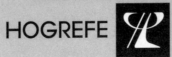